Student Work Manual for Introductory Clinical Pharmacology

Brenda
294 7308

STUDENT WORK MANUAL FOR INTRODUCTORY CLINICAL PHARMACOLOGY

Jeanne C. Scherer, RN, MS

formerly, Assistant Director, Medical-Surgical Coordinator and Instructor Sisters of Charity Hospital, School of Nursing, Buffalo, New York

FOURTH EDITION

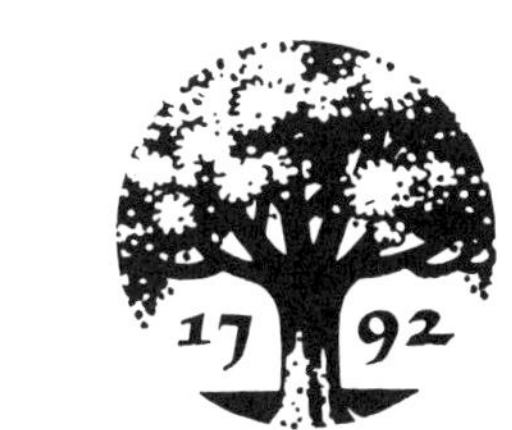

J.B. Lippincott Company
Philadelphia
New York, London, Hagerstown

Sponsoring Editor: Ellen Campbell
Production Manager: Lori J. Bainbridge
Editorial/Production: NB Enterprises
Compositor: Melissa Brown
Printer/Binder: Courier Westford

4th Edition

6 5 4

ISBN 0-397-54844-3

Any procedure or practice described in this book should be applied by the health care practitioner under appropriate supervision in accordance with professional standards of care used with regard to the unique circumstances that apply in each practice situation. Care has been taken to confirm the accuracy of information presented and to describe generally accepted practices. However, the authors, editors, and publisher cannot accept any responsibility for errors or omissions or for any consequences from application of the information in this book and make no warranty, express or implied, with respect to the contents of the book.

Every effort has been made to ensure drug selections and dosages are in accordance with current recommendations and practice. Because of ongoing research, changes in government regulations, and the constant flow of information on drug therapy, reactions, and interactions, the reader is cautioned to check the package insert for each drug for the indications, dosages, warnings, and precautions, particularly if the drug is new or infrequently used.

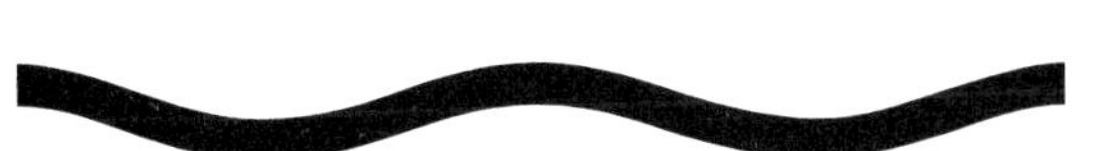

PREFACE

The *Student Work Manual* is designed to accompany the fourth edition of the textbook, *Introductory Clinical Pharmacology.* The purpose of this work manual is to provide a means of reviewing material as well as to furnish the student with practice in answering various types of test questions. *All* questions in this manual were constructed from the material contained in the textbook. The answers to each question are provided in the **Answers** section in the back of the book.

The first chapter of the textbook presents a review of arithmetic and the calculation of drug dosages. The manual has arithmetic drills and dosage calculation problems that are in the same order as the material presented in the textbook. The student may start with any section of the first chapter in the textbook or work manual depending on the extent of review or practice desired or needed. While many hospitals are using new medication delivery systems, some of which require that the preparation of individual medications by all routes be performed by a registered pharmacist, the nurse may, in certain situations, be required to perform dosage calculations.

The remaining chapters of the manual cover the material contained in the textbook. A variety of questions are included to give the user practice in answering a range of styles of test construction. Fill-in and essay questions are also provided which may be answered in the work manual or used as a focal point for classroom discussion.

JEANNE C. SCHERER, R.N., M.S.

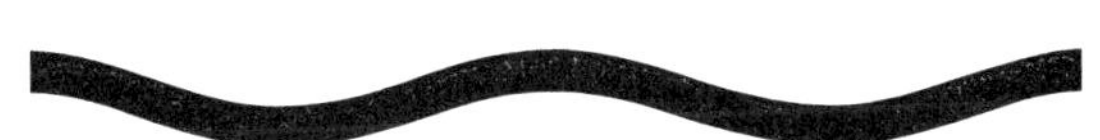

CONTENTS

A Review of Arithmetic and Calculation of Drug Dosages

The following list is provided to help you locate in the textbook the various topics covered in the questions in this chapter. These questions are based on the review of mathematical principles and the mathematics of pharmacology found in Chapter 1, **A Review of Arithmetic and Calculation of Drug Dosages**.

▶ ARITHMETIC REVIEW

▶ CALCULATION OF DRUG DOSAGES

▶ ARITHMETIC REVIEW

A. FRACTIONS

1. Name the two parts of a fraction.

_______________ _______________

2. Define the following.

a. Proper fraction _______________ b. Improper fraction _______________

3. In the blank provided, write the letters designating an *improper* fraction.

____

a. $\frac{7}{8}$	c. $\frac{9}{7}$	e. $\frac{2}{3}$	g. $\frac{4}{5}$	i. $\frac{2}{2}$
b. $\frac{5}{6}$	d. $\frac{1}{1}$	f. $\frac{5}{4}$	h. $\frac{4}{3}$	j. $\frac{9}{8}$

4. Briefly explain why the following is incorrectly expressed as a fraction?

$\frac{\text{2 grains}}{\text{7 ounces}}$ Explanation: _______________

B. MIXED NUMBERS AND IMPROPER FRACTIONS

1. What is a mixed number? _______________

2. Change the following mixed numbers to improper fractions.

a. $3\frac{3}{4}$ = ____	d. $1\frac{1}{3}$ = ____	g. $7\frac{1}{8}$ = ____	j. $5\frac{3}{4}$ = ____
b. $2\frac{1}{2}$ = ____	e. $5\frac{1}{2}$ = ____	h. $12\frac{2}{3}$ = ____	k. $3\frac{1}{3}$ = ____
c. $4\frac{1}{4}$ = ____	f. $8\frac{1}{2}$ = ____	i. $7\frac{1}{2}$ = ____	l. $20\frac{1}{3}$ = ____

3. Change the following improper fractions to mixed numbers.

a. $\frac{15}{4}$ = ____	d. $\frac{29}{4}$ = ____	g. $\frac{16}{5}$ = ____	j. $\frac{16}{3}$ = ____
b. $\frac{21}{4}$ = ____	e. $\frac{24}{5}$ = ____	h. $\frac{7}{6}$ = ____	k. $\frac{35}{4}$ = ____
c. $\frac{8}{3}$ = ____	f. $\frac{35}{3}$ = ____	i. $\frac{34}{5}$ = ____	l. $\frac{31}{2}$ = ____

C. ADDING FRACTIONS WITH LIKE DENOMINATORS

1. Add the following fractions and, when necessary, reduce the answer to the lowest possible terms.

a. $\frac{1}{8} + \frac{3}{8}$ = ____	f. $\frac{1}{5} + \frac{2}{5}$ = ____	k. $\frac{2}{3} + \frac{1}{3} + \frac{1}{3}$ = ____
b. $\frac{1}{4} + \frac{1}{4}$ = ____	g. $\frac{1}{2} + \frac{1}{2}$ = ____	l. $\frac{1}{4} + \frac{1}{4} + \frac{1}{4}$ = ____
c. $\frac{1}{6} + \frac{1}{6}$ = ____	h. $\frac{2}{7} + \frac{3}{7}$ = ____	m. $\frac{1}{10} + \frac{3}{10} + \frac{7}{10}$ = ____
d. $\frac{1}{3} + \frac{1}{3}$ = ____	i. $\frac{1}{8} + \frac{3}{8}$ = ____	
e. $\frac{5}{6} + \frac{1}{6}$ = ____	j. $\frac{3}{8} + \frac{3}{8}$ = ____	

2. Mr. Barnes is hired to plow 1/8 acre for one man and 3/8 acre for another man. How many total acres will Mr. Barnes plow? ______

3. For the present, disregard the terminology (ounces, cup, grain) in these problems and add the fractions.

a. $\frac{1}{2}$ ounce + $\frac{1}{2}$ ounce = ______

b. $\frac{1}{3}$ cup + $\frac{1}{3}$ cup = ______

c. $\frac{1}{4}$ cup + $\frac{1}{4}$ cup = ______

d. $\frac{1}{8}$ pound + $\frac{1}{8}$ pound = ______

e. $\frac{1}{32}$ ounce + $\frac{1}{32}$ ounce = ______

f. $\frac{1}{64}$ grain + $\frac{1}{64}$ grain = ______

g. You have 2 tablets of a drug and each tablet is 1/6 grain. If the 2 tablets are given together, how many grains of the drug are you giving? ______

D. ADDING FRACTIONS WITH UNLIKE DENOMINATORS

1. Add the following fractions and, when necessary, reduce to the answer to the lowest possible terms.

a. $\frac{2}{3} + \frac{1}{4} =$ ______

b. $\frac{1}{5} + \frac{1}{4} =$ ______

c. $\frac{1}{3} + \frac{1}{6} =$ ______

d. $\frac{1}{2} + \frac{1}{3} =$ ______

e. $\frac{1}{3} + \frac{1}{4} =$ ______

f. $\frac{4}{9} + \frac{1}{5} =$ ______

g. $\frac{1}{3} + \frac{1}{5} =$ ______

h. $\frac{1}{4} + \frac{2}{5} =$ ______

i. $\frac{1}{5} + \frac{3}{10} =$ ______

j. $\frac{2}{7} + \frac{1}{3} =$ ______

k. $\frac{1}{32} + \frac{1}{64} =$ ______

2. You have 2 containers. One weighs 1/4 pound and one weighs 1/6 pound. What is the total weight of the 2 containers in pounds? ______

3. Add the following fractions and change the improper fraction to a mixed number.

a. $\frac{1}{2} + \frac{2}{3} =$ ______

b. $\frac{2}{3} + \frac{5}{6} =$ ______

c. $\frac{1}{3} + \frac{8}{9} =$ ______

d. $\frac{4}{5} + \frac{2}{3} =$ ______

e. $\frac{3}{8} + \frac{9}{10} =$ ______

f. $\frac{6}{7} + \frac{2}{3} =$ ______

g. $\frac{10}{11} + \frac{1}{2} =$ ______

h. $\frac{3}{4} + \frac{7}{8} =$ ______

E. ADDING MIXED NUMBERS OR FRACTIONS AND MIXED NUMBERS

1. Add the following mixed numbers or fractions and mixed numbers.

a. $2\frac{1}{2} + 2\frac{1}{2} =$ ______

b. $1\frac{2}{3} + \frac{3}{4} =$ ______

c. $2\frac{2}{5} + 4\frac{1}{2} =$ ______

d. $3\frac{1}{3} + 2\frac{1}{3} =$ ______

e. $5\frac{1}{2} + \frac{1}{8} =$ ______

f. $7\frac{3}{4} + 7\frac{1}{2} =$ ______

g. $4\frac{1}{4} + \frac{2}{3} =$ ______

2. Again, disregard the terminology (ounces, pounds) used in these sample problems and concentrate on adding the fractions and mixed numbers.

a. $7\frac{1}{2}$ pounds + $7\frac{1}{2}$ pounds = ______

b. $3\frac{3}{4}$ pounds + $3\frac{3}{4}$ pounds = ______

c. $1\frac{1}{2}$ ounces + $3\frac{1}{4}$ ounces = ______

d. $1\frac{1}{2}$ pounds + $\frac{3}{4}$ pound = ______

e. $1\frac{1}{2}$ ounces + $1\frac{1}{2}$ ounces = ______

f. $1\frac{2}{3}$ ounces + $\frac{1}{2}$ ounce = ______

g. $\frac{1}{4}$ pound + $1\frac{1}{2}$ pounds = ______

F. COMPARISON OF FRACTIONS

1. Which is the largest fraction?

a. $\frac{1}{3}$ or $\frac{2}{3}$ ______ d. $\frac{3}{9}$ or $\frac{5}{9}$ ______ g. $\frac{1}{4}$ or $\frac{1}{2}$ ______ j. $\frac{2}{3}$ or $\frac{1}{2}$ ______

b. $\frac{5}{6}$ or $\frac{1}{6}$ ______ e. $\frac{2}{5}$ or $\frac{3}{5}$ ______ h. $\frac{3}{4}$ or $\frac{5}{8}$ ______ k. $\frac{5}{16}$ or $\frac{3}{8}$ ______

c. $\frac{1}{4}$ or $\frac{3}{4}$ ______ f. $\frac{2}{3}$ or $\frac{1}{10}$ ______ i. $\frac{2}{5}$ or $\frac{5}{9}$ ______ l. $\frac{2}{3}$ or $\frac{3}{5}$ ______

2. Mr. Burke receives 1/3 of the usual dose of a medicine, whereas Mr. Herman receives 1/6 of the usual dose of the same medicine. Which patient receives the larger dose? ______________

3. You read an older textbook which discusses drugs and their administration. The text states that the average dose of morphine is grain 1/6 to grain 1/4. Which is the larger of the two doses? ______________

G. MULTIPLYING FRACTIONS

1. Multiply the following fractions and, when necessary, reduce the answer to the lowest possible terms.

a. $\frac{1}{8} \times \frac{1}{4} =$ ______ d. $\frac{1}{2} \times \frac{2}{3} =$ ______ g. $\frac{4}{5} \times \frac{4}{5} =$ ______ j. $\frac{3}{4} \times \frac{1}{4} =$ ______

b. $\frac{1}{2} \times \frac{1}{2} =$ ______ e. $\frac{3}{5} \times \frac{1}{3} =$ ______ h. $\frac{4}{8} \times \frac{3}{6} =$ ______

c. $\frac{1}{3} \times \frac{2}{3} =$ ______ f. $\frac{7}{9} \times \frac{1}{3} =$ ______ i. $\frac{10}{12} \times \frac{2}{3} =$ ______

H. MULTIPLYING WHOLE NUMBERS AND FRACTIONS

1. Multiply the following whole numbers and fractions. When necessary, change the improper fraction of your answer to a mixed number and reduce to the lowest possible terms.

a. $5 \times \frac{1}{8} =$ ______ d. $3 \times \frac{1}{4} =$ ______ g. $2 \times \frac{3}{10} =$ ______ j. $4 \times \frac{1}{4} =$ ______

b. $4 \times \frac{2}{3} =$ ______ e. $5 \times \frac{1}{2} =$ ______ h. $7 \times \frac{2}{16} =$ ______ k. $7 \times \frac{6}{7} =$ ______

c. $1 \times \frac{1}{2} =$ ______ f. $7 \times \frac{1}{3} =$ ______ i. $3 \times \frac{2}{3} =$ ______ l. $2 \times \frac{1}{2} =$ ______

2. Two patients receive 500 mL of a dietary supplement. Mrs. Klein drank two thirds (2/3) of her supplement and Mrs. Cleary drank one half (1/2) of hers. Which patient drank more? ______________

I. MULTIPLYING MIXED NUMBERS

1. Multiply the following mixed numbers and, when necessary, reduce the answer to the lowest possible terms.

a. $2\frac{1}{2} \times 3\frac{1}{4} =$ ______ c. $4\frac{1}{4} \times 5\frac{1}{8} =$ ______ e. $2\frac{1}{4} \times 4\frac{1}{4} =$ ______ g. $1\frac{2}{3} \times 3\frac{1}{5} =$ ______

b. $3\frac{1}{2} \times 3\frac{1}{2} =$ ______ d. $1\frac{1}{2} \times 5\frac{6}{7} =$ ______ f. $5\frac{1}{4} \times 2\frac{1}{8} =$ ______ h. $2\frac{1}{6} \times 4\frac{1}{8} =$ ______

J. MULTIPLYING A WHOLE NUMBER AND A MIXED NUMBER

1. Multiply the following whole numbers and mixed numbers and, when necessary, reduce the answer to the lowest possible number.

a. $3 \times 2\frac{1}{2} =$ ______ c. $6 \times 1\frac{1}{2} =$ ______ e. $2 \times 4\frac{1}{4} =$ ______ g. $7 \times 2\frac{1}{4} =$ ______

b. $4 \times 3\frac{1}{2} =$ ______ d. $5 \times 5\frac{1}{4} =$ ______ f. $1 \times 3\frac{1}{3} =$ ______ h. $3 \times 4\frac{5}{8} =$ ______

2. Mr. Graham is to drink extra water. The glass he uses holds 8 ounces. He tells you he drank 2-1/2 glasses of water. How many ounces did he drink? ____________________

3. Mrs. Shields is to drink a protein supplement. Each container holds 3-1/2 ounces. She drank 3 containers in the past 5 hours. How many ounces of the protein supplement did Mrs. Shields drink? ____________________

4. Mr. Olcott received 1-1/2 bottles of intravenous fluid. Each bottle holds 500 milliliters. How many milliliters did Mr. Olcott receive? ____________________

5. Mrs. Best is admitted to the emergency room by ambulance. The examining physician tells you that Mrs. Best took 4 times the dose of the drug prescribed by her physician. If the directions on the drug container instructed her to take 2-1/2 tablets daily, how many tablets did Mrs. Best take? ____________________

K. DIVIDING FRACTIONS

1. Divide the following fractions and, when necessary, reduce the answer to the lowest possible terms.

a. $\frac{1}{8} \div \frac{1}{4} =$ ______	e. $\frac{1}{10} \div \frac{1}{2} =$ ______	i. $\frac{2}{3} \div \frac{1}{8} =$ ______	m. $\frac{1}{100} \div \frac{1}{1000} =$ ______
b. $\frac{1}{3} \div \frac{1}{2} =$ ______	f. $\frac{1}{7} \div \frac{2}{3} =$ ______	j. $\frac{2}{5} \div \frac{2}{3} =$ ______	n. $\frac{1}{250} \div \frac{1}{2} =$ ______
c. $\frac{1}{4} \div \frac{1}{6} =$ ______	g. $\frac{2}{3} \div \frac{1}{3} =$ ______	k. $\frac{3}{7} \div \frac{2}{3} =$ ______	o. $\frac{1}{100} \div \frac{1}{2} =$ ______
d. $\frac{1}{5} \div \frac{1}{12} =$ ______	h. $\frac{4}{5} \div \frac{1}{5} =$ ______	l. $\frac{5}{6} \div \frac{2}{3} =$ ______	p. $\frac{1}{100} \div \frac{1}{200} =$ ______

L. DIVIDING FRACTIONS AND MIXED NUMBERS

1. Divide the following fractions and mixed numbers and, when necessary, reduce the answer to the lowest possible terms.

a. $2\frac{1}{3} \div \frac{1}{4} =$ ______	c. $\frac{1}{2} \div 2\frac{1}{4} =$ ______	e. $\frac{1}{3} \div 1\frac{1}{4} =$ ______	g. $\frac{2}{3} \div 5\frac{3}{8} =$ ______
b. $2\frac{1}{2} \div \frac{1}{2} =$ ______	d. $1\frac{1}{2} \div \frac{2}{3} =$ ______	f. $3\frac{5}{8} \div \frac{4}{5} =$ ______	h. $\frac{1}{5} \div 2\frac{2}{3} =$ ______

2. Divide the following mixed numbers and, when necessary, reduce the answer to the lowest possible terms.

a. $1\frac{3}{4} \div 4\frac{1}{4} =$ ______	c. $2\frac{3}{4} \div 5\frac{1}{4} =$ ______	e. $6\frac{2}{3} \div 1\frac{1}{3} =$ ______	g. $1\frac{1}{2} \div 1\frac{1}{2} =$ ______
b. $1\frac{7}{8} \div 2\frac{1}{4} =$ ______	d. $8\frac{1}{2} \div 4\frac{1}{4} =$ ______	f. $5\frac{1}{2} \div 2\frac{2}{3} =$ ______	h. $9\frac{2}{3} \div 1\frac{1}{4} =$ ______

3. Divide the following whole numbers and fractions and, when necessary, reduce the answer to the lowest possible terms.

a. $2 \div \frac{2}{3} =$ ______	d. $\frac{1}{3} \div 2 =$ ______	g. $\frac{1}{32} \div 2 =$ ______	j. $\frac{1}{8} \div 2 =$ ______
b. $\frac{1}{4} \div 2 =$ ______	e. $\frac{2}{3} \div 2 =$ ______	h. $\frac{1}{2} \div 2 =$ ______	
c. $4 \div \frac{1}{4} =$ ______	f. $6 \div \frac{1}{4} =$ ______	i. $\frac{1}{16} \div 2 =$ ______	

4. Divide the following whole numbers and mixed numbers and, when necessary, reduce the answer to the lowest possible terms.

a. $4 \div 2\frac{2}{3} =$ ______	c. $6 \div 2\frac{1}{4} =$ ______	e. $2\frac{1}{2} \div 2 =$ ______
b. $2 \div 1\frac{1}{2} =$ ______	d. $3\frac{1}{3} \div 4 =$ ______	f. $4\frac{1}{2} \div 5 =$ ______

M. RATIO

1. Define a ratio. ______________________________

____

2. Write the following both as a ratio and as a fraction. When necessary, reduce to the lowest possible terms.

	Ratio	Fraction
a. one part to ten parts	________	________
b. two parts to fifteen parts	________	________
c. five parts to twenty-five parts	________	________
d. one part to one hundred parts	________	________
e. one part to two hundred fifty parts	________	________

3. Write the following ratios as fractions.

a. 1:1000 = ______ c. 1:6 = ______ e. 1:2 = ______

b. 1:50 = ______ d. 2:3 = ______

4. Express the following fractions as ratios.

a. $\frac{1}{4}$ = ______ c. $\frac{1}{32}$ = ______

b. $\frac{1}{150}$ = ______ d. $\frac{1}{5000}$ = ______

5. If one man owns 1/4 acre and another man owns 1/2 acre, which is the largest piece of land?

____

6. If one solution is labeled 1/4 strength and another solution labeled 1/2 strength, which is the stronger solution?

____

7. If a solution is labeled 1:5000, is it stronger or weaker than a solution labeled 1:500? ______________
8. If one drug is 1/64 grain and another drug is 1/32 grain, which is the weaker drug? ______________

N. PERCENT

1. What does the term percent mean? ______________________________

____

2. Express each of the following percent as parts per hundred.

a. 32% ______ c. 40% ______ e. 20% ______

b. 64% ______ d. 90% ______

3. Mary received 84% on her history test. If there were 100 questions on the test, how many were correct?

____

Express Mary's grade as parts per hundred. ______________

Express Mary's grade as a fraction. ______________

4. Change each of the following percents to a fraction and, when necessary, reduce the answer to the lowest possible terms.

a. 25% ______ c. 37% ______ e. 41% ______ g. 84% ______

b. 50% ______ d. 75% ______ f. 22% ______ h. 90% ______

5. Change each of the following fractions to a percent.

a. $\frac{4}{5}$ = ______ d. $\frac{5}{8}$ = ______ g. $\frac{3}{8}$ = ______ j. $\frac{1}{10}$ = ______

b. $\frac{1}{2}$ = ______ e. $\frac{2}{5}$ = ______ h. $\frac{1}{4}$ = ______

c. $\frac{2}{3}$ = ______ f. $\frac{1}{7}$ = ______ i. $\frac{1}{6}$ = ______

6. Change each of the following ratios to a percent.

a. 1:500 = _______ d. 1:8 = _______ g. 1:4 = _______ j. 1:200 = _______

b. 1:100 = _______ e. 1:25 = _______ h. 1:10 = _______

c. 1:1000 = _______ f. 1:5000 = _______ i. 1:2000 = _______

7. Change each of the following percents to a ratio.

a. 5% _______ c. 30% _______ e. 1% _______ g. 8% _______

b. 25% _______ d. 80% _______ f. 0.3% _______ h. 12% _______

8. Jack claims he can beat his golf partner 1 out of 5 times. Express Jack's winning at golf as a ratio ____________________, as a fraction ____________________, and as a percent ____________________.

9. Mrs. Conrad has a solution applied to her leg ulcer. The bottle is labeled 1:250. What is the percent of the solution? ____________________

10. A solution used for bladder irrigations is labeled 1:4000. What is the percentage of the solution? ____________________

11. Mr. Jennings has an irrigating solution labeled 10%. Express 10% as a ratio. ____________________

O. PROPORTION

1. Solve the following problems for x.

a. 5:10::10:x x = _______

b. $3/x = 5/20$ x = _______

c. 2:6 as x:9 x = _______

d. 1:7::10:x x = _______

e. $15/1 = 30/x$ x = _______

f. 6:12::x:144 x = _______

2. Set up and solve the following proportions.

a. If a man takes 15 hours to pick all the corn planted on one acre, how many acres can he pick in 30 hours?

Proportion: ____________________

Solution: x = _______ acres.

b. Using the same figures but substituting medical terminology, if 15 grains equals 1 gram, how many grams are in 30 grains?

Proportion: ____________________

Solution: x = _______ grains.

c. If you could buy 2.2 yards of ribbon for one dollar, how many yards of ribbon could you buy for forty dollars?

Proportion: ____________________

Solution: x = _______ yards.

d. Using the same figures but substituting medical terminology, if 2.2 pounds equals 1 kilogram, how many pounds are in 40 kilograms?

Proportion: ____________________

Solution: x = _______ pounds

e. If one share of a stock went up 1/60 of a dollar, how many dollars would you make on 6 shares of stock?

Proportion: ____________________

Solution: x = _______

f. Using the same figures but substituting medical terminology, if 1 milligram equals 1/60 of a grain, how many grains are there in 6 milligrams?

Proportion: ____________________

Solution: x = _______

g. If 30 milligrams equals 1/2 grain, how many grains are in 90 milligrams?

Proportion: ____________________

Solution: x = _______

h. If 5 milligrams of a drug is given for every kilogram of body weight, how much of the drug is given to the patient weighing 64 kilograms?

Proportion: ____________________

Solution: x = _______

P. DECIMALS

1. What is a decimal? ______________________________

____

2. Both decimal fractions and mixed decimal fractions are commonly referred to as decimals.

   a. What is a decimal fraction? ______________________________

   ____

   b. What is a mixed decimal? ______________________________

   ____

3. Place an X on the line identifying the following decimals.

	Decimal Fraction	**Mixed Decimal**
a. 0.01	________	________
b. 1.45	________	________
c. 0.33	________	________
d. 2.5	________	________
e. 7.5	________	________
f. 0.45	________	________
g. 1.25	________	________

4. Write the following as decimals.

   a. nine tenths ________

   b. four hundredths ________

   c. five and four tenths ________

   d. one tenth ________

   e. two hundredths ________

   f. one thousandth ________

5. Write out the following decimals.

   a. 0.4 is read as ________

   b. 0.75 is read as ________

   c. 1.6 is read as ________

   d. 5.58 is read as ________

   e. 7.755 is read as ________

6. Add the following decimals.

   a. $2.25 + 5.86 =$ ______

   b. $3.75 + 0.66 =$ ______

   c. $1.75 + 2.25 =$ ______

   d. $23.65 + 0.56 =$ ______

   e. $475.45 + 4.66 =$ ______

   f. $62.32 + 0.007 =$ ______

   g. $5.63 + 4.24 + 3.1 =$ ______

   h. $66.2 + 0.25 + 1.755 =$ ______

7. Subtract the following decimals.

   a. $5.5 - 3.4 =$ ______

   b. $68.07 - 14.6 =$ ______

   c. $1.77 - 0.015 =$ ______

   d. $7.75 - 3.875 =$ ______

8. Multiply the following whole numbers and decimals.

   a. $5 \times 0.5 =$ ______

   b. $25 \times 0.1 =$ ______

   c. $2 \times 2.25 =$ ______

   d. $15 \times 1.4 =$ ______

9. Multiply the following decimals.

   a. $2.75 \times 0.5 =$ ______

   b. $4.4 \times 1.2 =$ ______

   c. $2.5 \times 2.5 =$ ______

   d. $6.25 \times 1.15 =$ ______

   e. $7.5 \times 2.5 =$ ______

   f. $1.5 \times 1.5 =$ ______

   g. $5.46 \times 2.17 =$ ______

   h. $1.5 \times 3.5 =$ ______

10. Divide the following decimals.

a. 0.65 ÷ 0.3 = _______
b. 0.7 ÷ 0.2 = _______
c. 1.42 ÷ 0.62 = _______
d. 4 ÷ 0.75 = _______
e. 6 ÷ 2.2 = _______
f. 5 ÷ 5.5 = _______
g. 4.4 ÷ 3 = _______
h. 3.6 ÷ 2 = _______

11. Change each of the following decimals to a fraction and, when necessary, reduce the answer to the lowest possible terms.

a. 0.2 = _______
b. 0.65 = _______
c. 0.87 = _______
d. 0.5 = _______
e. 0.68 = _______

▶ THE CALCULATION OF DRUG DOSAGES

A. SYSTEMS OF MEASUREMENT

1. Name the three systems of measurement.

a. _______________ b. _______________ c. _______________

2. Which system is most commonly used for the dosage of drugs? _______________

3. The unit of weight in the metric system is the _______________.

4. The unit of volume in the metric system is the _______________.

5. The unit of length in the metric system is the _______________.

6. The units of weight in the apothecaries' system are _______________, _______________, and _______________.

7. The units of volume in the apothecaries' system are _______________, _______________, and _______________.

8. Write the abbreviations or symbols for the following.

a. milligram _______________
b. kilogram _______________
c. nanogram _______________
d. microgram _______________
e. liter _______________
f. milliliter _______________
g. centimeter _______________
h. meter _______________
i. grain _______________
j. minims (symbol) _______________

B. CONVERSIONS BETWEEN SYSTEMS

1. Although the apothecaries' system is rarely used today, nurses may, on occasion, need to use this system. A few problems requiring conversion between the metric and apothecaries' have been included for practice in conversion between these two systems. Convert the following. Label the answer with the correct abbreviation.

a. 30 grains to grams ________
b. 4.4 pounds to kilograms ________
c. 66 pounds to kilograms ________
d. 2 milligrams to grains ________
e. 8 minims to milliliters ________
f. 1 quart to liters ________
g. 2 fluid ounces to milliliters ________
h. 1-1/2 grains to grams ________
i. 1 quart to milliliters ________
j. 1/100 grain to milligrams ________
k. 1 milligram to micrograms ________
l. 1/4 grain to milligrams ________
m. 15 minims to milliliters ________
n. 500 milliliters to pints ________
o. 30 minims to milliliters ________
p. 60 grains to grams ________
q. 1/60 grain to milligrams ________

2. Some drug dosages are based on the patient's weight. Convert the following. Label the answer with the correct abbreviation.

a. 55 pounds to kilograms ________
b. 140 pounds to kilograms ________
c. 86 kilograms to pounds ________
d. 52 kilograms to pounds ________
e. 156 pounds to kilograms ________
f. 126 pounds to kilograms ________

C. CONVERTING WITHIN A SYSTEM

1. Convert the following metric measurements. Label the answer with the correct abbreviation.

a. 2000 mL to liters ________
b. 60 mg to grams ________
c. 1.5 g to milligrams ________
d. 0.1 g to milligrams ________
e. 3000 mL to liters ________
f. 0.5 g to milligrams ________
g. 750 mg to grams ________
h. 2000 mcg to milligrams ________
i. 0.2 mg to micrograms ________
j. 500 mL to liters ________
k. 1500 mL to liters ________
l. 500 mg to grams ________
m. 2.5 g to milligrams ________
n. 100 mg to grams ________
o. 500 mcg to milligrams ________
p. 1.5 L to milliliters ________

D. ORAL DOSAGES OF DRUGS

1. Using D/H = x or any other method, find the correct dosage of the following solid oral preparations. Label each numerical answer correctly, as example 2 *tablets*, 1 *capsule* and so on.

a. Ordered: codeine sulfate 60 mg.
Have available: codeine sulfate 30-mg tablets
Give: ________

b. Ordered: ampicillin 0.5 g
Have available: ampicillin 250-mg capsules
Give: ________

c. Ordered: phenobarbital gr 1/4
Have available: phenobarbital 15-mg tablets
Give: ________

d. Ordered: Chloromycetin 0.25 g
Have available: Chloromycetin 250-mg capsules
Give: ________

e. Ordered: papaverine 0.1 g
Have available: papaverine 100-mg tablets
Give: ________

f. Ordered: nylidrin 12 mg
Have available: nylidrin 6-mg tablets
Give: ________

g. Ordered: Seconal 0.1 g
Have available: Seconal 100-mg capsules
Give: ____________

h. Ordered: Tapazole 15 mg
Have available: Tapazole 5-mg tablets
Give: ____________

i. Ordered: glutethimide 500 mg
Have available: glutethimide 0.5-g tablets
Give: ____________

j. Ordered: Gemonil 50 mg
Have available: Gemonil 100-mg tablets
Give: ____________

k. Ordered: warfarin 5 mg
Have available: warfarin 2.5-mg tablets
Give: ____________

2. Using proportion or any other method, answer the following questions. Note that some of these problems may require a conversion within a system before or after the problem is solved.

a. If the total daily dose of a drug is 0.9 g and the drug is given in three equally divided doses each day, what is the amount of each dose in *milligrams*? ____________

b. If the dose of a drug is 10 mg for each kilogram of body weight, what is the dose for an adult weighing 132 pounds? ____________

c. If the dose of a drug is 2.5 mg for each kilogram of body weight, what is the dose for a child weighing 44 pounds? ____________

d. The total daily dose of a drug is 1 g and is to be divided into four equal doses. How many milligrams are in each dose? ____________

e. If a drug is available as 250-mg tablets and 0.5 g are given bid (twice a day), what is the total number of tablets given each day?
____

3. Using D/H × Q = *x* or any other method, find the correct dosage of the following liquid oral preparations. Label each numerical answer correctly.

a. Ordered: erythromycin 200 mg
Have available: erythromycin syrup 100 mg/2.5 mL
Give: ____________

b. Ordered: Paradione 600 mg
Have available: Paradione 300 mg/mL
Give: ____________

c. Ordered: Amcill 250 mg
Have available: Amcill 125 mg/5 mL
Give: ____________

d. Ordered: potassium chloride 20 mEq
Have available: potassium chloride 40 mEq/15 mL
Give: ____________

e. Ordered: NegGram 125 mg
Have available: NegGram 0.25 g/5 mL
Give: ____________

f. Ordered: Dilantin 0.25 g
Have available: Dilantin 125 mg/5 mL
Give: ____________

E. PARENTERAL DOSAGES OF DRUGS

1. Using D/H × Q = *x* or any other method, determine the correct dosage for the following parenteral preparations. These problems also illustrate some of the labeling and written variations that may be found in clinical practice. Label each numerical answer correctly, as example, *mL*, *mcg*, and so on.

a. Ordered: Demerol 75 mg
Have available: Demerol 50 mg/mL
Give: ____________

b. Ordered: Valium 5 mg
Have available: Valium 10 mg/2 mL
Give: ____________

c. Ordered: atropine sulfate gr 1/200
Have available: atropine sulfate 0.3 mg/mL
Give: ____________

d. Ordered: Kantrex 37.5 mg
Have available: Kantrex 75 mg/2 mL
Give: ____________

e. Ordered: Stadol 1 mg
Have available: Stadol 2 mg/mL
Give: ____________

f. Ordered: digoxin 0.25 mg
Have available: digoxin 0.5 mg/2 mL
Give: ____________

g. Ordered: digoxin 0.125 mg
Have available: digoxin 0.5 mg/2 mL
Give: ____________

h. Ordered: Apresoline 40 mg
Have available: Apresoline 20 mg/mL
Give: ____________

i. Ordered: Neo-Synephrine 5 mg
Have available: Neo-Synephrine 1% (10 mg/mL)
Give: ____________

j. Ordered: Desferal 0.5 g
Have available: deferoxamine 500 mg/2 mL
Give: ____________

k. Ordered: Priscoline 50 mg
   Have available: Priscoline 4 mL ampule labeled 1 mL = 25 mg
   Give: 2 ml

l. Ordered: fentanyl 0.1 mg
   Have available: fentanyl 0.05 mg/mL
   Give: 2 ml

m. Ordered: Duracillin 150,000 units
   Have available: Duracillin 300,000 U/mL
   Give: .5 mL

The stronger the strength the smaller the amounts

n. The dose of Mithracin, based on the patient's weight, is 25 mcg/kg. Mithracin is available as 500 mcg/mL when diluted according to the manufacturer's directions. The patient weighs 110 pounds. How many milliliters are given to this patient? 2.5 ml

o. Ordered: heparin 5000 units
   Have available: heparin 2500 U/mL
   Give: 2 ml

p. Ordered: Keflin 500 mg
   Have available: Keflin 1 g/10 mL
   Give: 5 ml

2. Drugs in dry form must be made into a liquid (reconstitution) before they are administered. Directions for reconstitution are usually printed on the label or included in the package insert. Using D/H × Q = *x* or any other method, determine the volume given for the prescribed dosage. The manufacturer's directions are included in each problem. Label each numerical answer in *milliliters*.

a. Ordered: Pipracil 3 g IV piggyback
   Have available: Pipracil 4-g vial in powder form
   Directions for reconstitution: reconstitute each gram with 2 mL of any of the recommended diluents listed in the package insert to make 1 g per 2.5 mL
   Give: 7.5 mL

b. Ordered: Ticar 1 g IM
   Have available: 6-g Ticar vial in powder form
   Directions for reconstitution: add 2 mL of sodium chloride for each gram. Each 2.5 mL of solution will equal 1 g.
   Give: 2.5 ml

c. A vial of penicillin G aqueous is labeled as follows: 5,000,000 units per vial. A vial may be reconstituted with 23 mL, 18 mL, 8 mL, or 3 mL to provide 200,000 U, 250,000 U, 500,000 U, or 1 million U per mL, respectively. Answer the following questions regarding this drug.

   1. If the physician orders 1,000,000 U to be given, how much diluent would you use to provide 1,000,000 units/mL?
      3 ml.
   2. If you dilute the 5,000,000-U vial with 23 mL, how many units of penicillin are in each milliliter? 200,000 U
   3. If the physician ordered 500,000 U to be given IM, what amount of diluent is added to the vial to give 500,000 U/mL?
      8 mL

23 ml = 200,000 u/ml
18 ml = 250,000 u/ml
8 ml = 500,000 u/ml
3 ml = 1,000,000 u/ml

d. Ordered: Azlin 1.5 g IV piggyback
   Have available: Azlin 2-g vial
   Directions for reconstitution: add 10 mL of any one of the diluents reommended in the package insert to make 2 g/10 mL
   Give: 7.5 ml

F. TEMPERATURES

1. Convert the following temperatures written in Fahrenheit to Celsius.

a. 98.6° F = ______
b. 100° F = ______
c. 101° F = ______
d. 101.4° F = ______
e. 97° F = ______

2. Convert the following temperatures written in Celsius to Fahrenheit.

a. 36.2° C = ______
b. 30° C = ______
c. 38.4° C = ______
d. 38° C = ______

G. PEDIATRIC DOSAGES

1. The physician orders Staphcillin by IV infusion for a child weighing 32 pounds. Literature states that the pediatric dose is 100 to 300 mg/kg/day in divided doses. The drug is ordered to be given every 4 hours.
   a. Convert the child's weight of 32 pounds to kilograms. ____________
   b. Compute the total daily dose for a child weighing 32 pounds based on a dose of 100 mg/kg/day. ____________
   c. How many times per day is the drug given? ____________
   d. How many milligrams are given each dose? ____________
2. The recommended pediatric dose of Dilantin is 5 mg/kg/day in 2 or 3 equally divided doses.
   a. What is the total daily dose for a child weighing 30 kilograms? ____________
   b. If the drug is ordered 3 times/day, how many milligrams are given each dose? ____________
   c. The drug is available as Dilantin-30 Pediatric at 30 mg/5 mL. How many milliliters are given in each dose? ____________
3. The recommended total IV digitalizing dose of digoxin for a child 5 to 10 years of age is 15 to 30 mcg/kg.
   a. What is the weight, in kilograms, of a child weighing 72 pounds? ____________
   b. What is the IV digitalizing dose range, in micrograms (mcg), for a child weighing 72 pounds? ____________
   c. How many micrograms are there in one milligram? ____________
4. Body Surface Area (BSA)

$$\frac{\text{Surface area of child in square meters}}{\text{Surface area of adult in square meters (1.7)}} \times \text{usual adult dose} = \text{child dose}$$

If the BSA of a child is 0.4 square meters (m^2), the BSA of an adult is 1.7 square meters (m^2), and the average adult dose of a drug is 100 mg, what is the child dose of the drug? ____________

H. SOLUTIONS

1. What is a solute? ____
2. Most solutions requiring preparation before use are prepared by a hospital pharmacist. On occasion, such as in an emergency or disaster, the nurse may find it necessary to prepare a solution before use. Using proportion or any other method, prepare the following solution.
   Strength of solution on hand: 100%
   Strength of solution desired: 20%
   Amount of solution desired: 2000 mL

   How many milliliters of the 100% solution will be needed to make 2000 mL of a 20% solution? ____________

   How many milliliters would be required to make 1000 mL of a 20% solution? ____________
3. Strength of drug on hand: 4-gram tablets
   Strength of solution desired: 8%
   Amount of solution desired: 100 mL

   How many 4-gram tablets are required to make 100 mL of an 8% solution? ____________

   How many tablets would be required to make a 20% solution? ____________

2

The Administration of Medications

The following questions are concerned with the contents of Chapter 2, **The Administration of Medications**.

I. FILL-IN AND ESSAY QUESTIONS

Read each question carefully and place your answer in the space provided.

1. List or describe the five rights in the administration of drugs.

   ____

   ____

   ____

   ____

   ____

2. A physician's written order is necessary for the administration of all drugs. What situation may be an exception to this rule?

   ____

3. When preparing a drug for administration the label is checked three times. List or describe the times at which the label of the drug is checked.

   First time ______________________________

   Second time ______________________________

   Third time ______________________________

4. What is the most frequent route of drug administration?

   ____

5. Briefly explain why the patient should be placed in an upright position when receiving an oral drug.

   ____

   ____

6. Briefly explain why water is taken after an oral drug is swallowed.

____

____

____

7. Name any three parenteral administration routes.

   1. ____

   2. ____

   3. ____

8. When a drug is given by the intra-articular route it is given into what structure?

____

9. Answer yes or no. Is it normal to see blood appear when pulling back on the syringe barrel prior to giving an intramuscular injection? ______________; an intravenous injection? ______________.

10. A subcutaneous injection places the drug between which two structures?

______________ and ______________

11. A subcutaneous injection is given at a ______ degree angle and an intramuscular injection at a ______ degree angle.

12. When is the Z-track technique used to give a drug by the intramuscular route?

____

____

13. How soon does a drug take effect when it is given intravenously?

____

14. When giving a drug intravenously, is the tourniquet placed above or below the selected site of venipuncture? ____________________

15. True or false: Most topical drugs are not absorbed through the skin. ______________

16. Name any four of the various forms of topical application.

   1. ____

   2. ____

   3. ____

   4. ____

17. List any two nursing responsibilities following the administration of a drug.

   1. ____

   2. ____

II. CALCULATING IV FLOW RATES

1. Using any method, calculate the following IV flow rates:

   a. 1000 mL to infuse in 8 hours. The drop factor is 14. The IV solution should infuse at ________ drops per minute.

   b. 500 mL to infuse in 6 hours. The drop factor is 14. The IV solution should infuse at ________ drops per minute.

   c. 1000 mL to infuse in 6 hours. The drop factor is 12. The IV solution should infuse at ________ drops per minute.

3

General Principles of Pharmacology

The following questions are concerned with the contents of Chapter 3, **General Principles of Pharmacology**.

I. TRUE OR FALSE

Read each statement carefully and place your answer in the space provided.

1. ______ The age of a patient may influence the action of a drug.
2. ______ Only dosages for children are calculated on a weight basis.
3. ______ Women may require a smaller dosage of a drug than men.
4. ______ Certain diseases may require a reduction in the dosage of a drug.
5. ______ The most rapid drug action is produced by intramuscular administration.
6. ______ The ingestion of food may impair the absorption of a drug.
7. ______ A cumulative drug effect may be seen in the patient with severe kidney disease.

II. MULTIPLE CHOICE QUESTIONS

Circle the letter of the most appropriate answer.

1. Liver disease may result in a(n) _______.
   a. increase in the excretion rate of a drug
   b. impaired ability to metabolize or detoxify a drug
   c. necessity to increase the dosage of a drug
   d. decrease in the rate of drug absorption
2. The slowest drug action is usually produced when a drug is given _______.
   a. orally
   b. intramuscularly
   c. intravenously
   d. subcutaneously
3. An antagonistic drug effect may be defined as a(n) _______.
   a. increased drug effect
   b. neutralizing drug effect
   c. opposite drug effect
   d. repeat in drug action
4. A synergistic drug effect may be defined as a(n) _______.
   a. effect greater than the sum of the separate actions of two or more drugs
   b. increase in the action of one of the two drugs being given
   c. neutralizing drug effect
   d. comprehensive drug effect

5. When a drug is taken on an empty stomach it will be _______.
   a. absorbed more slowly
   b. neutralized by pancreatic enzymes
   c. affected by enzymes in the colon
   d. absorbed more rapidly
6. Adverse drug reactions _______.
   a. only occur when large doses of a drug are given
   b. may occur without warning
   c. are mild and should cause no concern
   d. are seen rarely in healthy individuals
7. Drug allergy is also called a(n) _______.
   a. synergistic reaction
   b. antagonistic effect
   c. drug idiosyncrasy
   d. hypersensitivity reaction
8. Allergic drug reactions _______.
   a. may be manifested by a variety of signs and symptoms
   b. occur when the patient produces antigens
   c. are predictable
   d. usually occur only after the drug is discontinued
9. An anaphylactic drug reaction is characterized by _______.
   a. hypertension, cyanosis, bradycardia
   b. tachycardia, decreased respiratory rate, dyspnea
   c. bronchospasm, hypotension, loss of consciousness
   d. anxiety, hypertension, cardiac dysrhythmias
10. Drug idiosyncrasy is a term used to describe _______.
    a. an expected drug response
    b. any unusual or abnormal reaction to a drug
    c. drug activity in elderly patients
    d. an allergic drug reaction
11. Drug tolerance is a term used to describe a(n) _______.
    a. decreased response to a drug; usually necessitates an increase in dosage to give the desired effect
    b. inability of the patient to take a medication
    c. allergic drug reaction
    d. increased response to an average dose of a drug
12. A cumulative drug effect occurs when _______.
    a. an overdose of a drug is given accidentally
    b. a drug is excreted too rapidly
    c. a drug is given with food
    d. the body is unable to metabolize normally and excrete a drug
13. If a narcotic is classed as a Schedule II (C-II) drug it _______.
    a. has very little abuse potential
    b. has no accepted medical use
    c. has high abuse potential with severe dependence liability
    d. can only be dispensed to those with a terminal illness
14. The use of any medication, prescription or nonprescription, carries a risk of causing birth defects in the developing fetus. A drug or substance considered to be least likely to harm the developing fetus is labeled as Pregnancy Category _______.
    a. a   b. b   c. c   d. x

III. FILL-IN AND ESSAY QUESTIONS

Read each question carefully and place your answer in the space provided.

1. Briefly describe the purpose of the Pure Food, Drug and Cosmetic Act of 1938.

   ____

   ____

2. What is regulated by the Comprehensive Drug Abuse Prevention and Controlled Substances Act of 1978?

   ____

   ____

3. Determine the drug dosages for the following patients.
   a. Drug dosage: 5 mg/kg/day in two equally divided doses. Weight of patient: 120 pounds. Each dose will be _______ mg
   b. Drug dosage: 2 mg/kg/day in three equally divided doses. Weight of patient: 70 kg. Each dose will be _______ mg
   c. Drug dosage: 10 mg/kg/day in four equally divided doses. Weight of patient: 80 kg. Each dose will be _______ mg

The Nursing Process and the Administration of Pharmacologic Agents

The following questions are concerned with the contents of Chapter 4, **The Nursing Process and the Administration of Pharmacologic Agents**.

I. FILL-IN AND ESSAY QUESTIONS

Read each question carefully and place your answer in the space provided.

1. List the five parts of the nursing process.
   1. Assesment
   2. Nursing diagnosis
   3. Planning
   4. Implemention
   5. Evaluation
2. Give one reason why data obtained during assessment are an important aspect of drug administration. It provides data base, identifies problems, may influence decision in planning
3. Define **objective** data. are information obtained during physical assessment
4. Define **subjective** data. are data given to the nurse by the client or its family

5. Briefly explain the purpose of formulating a nursing diagnosis.

to identify problems that can be solved or prevented by means of independent nursing actions

6. Briefly explain what is involved in planning when it is part of the nursing process.

sorting and analyzing data
development of patient care plan, setting goals
plan steps for carrying out nursing activities

7. Briefly explain what is involved in implementation when it is part of the nursing process.

carry out the plan of action

8. When applied to pharmacology, implementation involves which nursing activities?

preparation and administering of the drug

9. When related to the administration of pharmacologic agents, evaluation may be defined or described as

The patient response to the drug.

5

Patient and Family Teaching

The following questions are concerned with the contents of Chapter 5, **Patient and Family Teaching**.

I. TRUE OR FALSE

Read each statement carefully and place your answer in the space provided.

1. __T__ Medical terminology is avoided when teaching the patient or a family member.
2. __F__ Patient teaching is best completed in one session, even when much material is presented.
3. __T__ Patient teaching plans must be individualized.
4. __F__ The term "drug" applies only to prescription drugs.
5. __F__ If a dose of a drug is omitted because the patient forgot to take the drug, she/he should be advised to double the next dose.

II. MULTIPLE CHOICE QUESTIONS

Circle the letter of the most appropriate answer.

1. If a drug changes color or develops a new odor _______.
   a. the drug should be placed in a different container
   b. a pharmacist should be asked about continued use of the drug
   c. the drug should be refrigerated for several days
   d. this is a normal chemical change in the drug
2. Two or more different drugs _______.
   a. should never be mixed in the same container
   b. can be placed in the same container
3. Drugs should not be exposed to heat, sunlight, cold, or moisture because _______.
   a. they may change color
   b. a poisonous residue may be left in the container
   c. one drug may chemically affect another
   d. the printing on the label may fade
4. Unless the physician or pharmacist directs otherwise, patients should be told to take oral medications with _______.
   a. fruit juice b. milk c. water d. food
5. If a patient is prescribed colored tablets and asks if they can be chewed before swallowing, your best response would be that _______.
   a. any tablet can be chewed
   b. tablets are never chewed
   c. only drugs labeled as chewable should be chewed
   d. only white tablets can be chewed

6. Mr. Billings tells you that the antibiotic prescribed for him is to be taken for 2 weeks. After 6 days his symptoms are gone and he asks if he can stop taking the drug. The best response would be _______.

   a. do not stop taking the drug unless advised to do so by the physician
   b. stop taking the drug and call the physician
   c. check with a pharmacist about stopping the drug
   d. stop the drug and mention this to the physician at the time of the next office visit

III. FILL-IN AND ESSAY QUESTIONS

Read each question carefully and place your answer in the space provided.

1. Briefly explain how the assessment part of the nursing process is used to develop a patient teaching plan.

   The data collected on assessment helps to determine the client's ability to learn, accepts and used information

2. Briefly describe some of the information you would like to know if you were prescribed a drug.

   The route to take it.
   The adverse effect.
   The time & frequency.
   If it would be best to be taken on an empty stomach versus full.

6

Adrenergic Drugs

The following questions are concerned with the contents of Chapter 6, **Adrenergic Drugs**.

I. TRUE OR FALSE

Read each statement carefully and place your answer in the space provided.

1. ______ The nervous system is concerned with the regulation and coordination of body activities.
2. ______ The central nervous system (CNS) consists of the brain and peripheral nerves.
3. ______ The somatic part of the peripheral nervous system is concerned with involuntary movement.
4. ______ The autonomic nervous system is concerned with functions essential to survival of the organism.
5. ______ Adrenergic drugs act like or mimic the activity of the sympathetic nervous system.
6. ______ Adrenergic drugs may produce sleepiness and slowed reactions to stimuli.
7. ______ Adrenergic drugs increase the heart rate.
8. ______ An adrenergic drug may be applied topically for the relief of nasal congestion.
9. ______ Adverse reactions associated with adrenergic drugs may depend on the drug used and the dose administered.
10. ______ A common adverse reaction associated with adrenergic drugs is a drop in blood pressure.

II. MULTIPLE CHOICE QUESTIONS

Circle the letter of the most appropriate answer.

1. The autonomic nervous system consists of the ______.
   a. brain and spinal cord
   b. somatic and asomatic nervous systems
   c. sympathetic and parasympathetic nervous systems
   d. nerves concerned with voluntary movement
2. The voluntary part of the somatic nervous system is concerned with ______.
   a. voluntary movement of skeletal muscles
   b. digestion of food
   c. voluntary movement of smooth muscles
   d. the heart and respiratory rate
3. The parasympathetic nervous system ______.
   a. controls the activity of skeletal muscles
   b. is operative when the organism is in danger
   c. is under the control of higher nerve centers in the brain
   d. works to help conserve body energy
4. Two neurohormones (or neurotransmitters) of the sympathetic nervous system are ______.
   a. epinephrine and norepinephrine
   b. acetylcholine and acetylcholinesterase
   c. epinephrine and ephedrine
   d. dopamine and levodopamine

5. Which of the following responses may be produced by an adrenergic drug? _______
   a. decrease in heart rate
   b. relaxation of the bronchi
   c. conservation of glucose
   d. dilatation of blood vessels
6. Which of the following are uses of adrenergic drugs? _______
   1. the management of cardiac arrest
   2. treatment of some ventricular dysrhythmias
   3. the treatment of hypertension
   4. temporary treatment of heart block

   a. 1, 2, 3 b. 1, 2, 4 c. 1, 4 d. all of these
7. Some of the more common adverse reactions seen with the administration of adrenergic drugs include _______.
   a. bradycardia, hypotension, bronchial constriction
   b. increase in appetite, nervousness, drowsiness
   c. nausea, vomiting, hypotension
   d. cardiac dysrhythmias, increase in blood pressure, headache
8. Assessment of the patient receiving an adrenergic drug will depend on the _______.
   a. nurse's ability to perform an assessment
   b. dose to be given
   c. drug, patient, and reason for administration
   d. patient's allergy history

Clinical Situation

Mr. Alden is in shock, and the physician has ordered norepinephrine, a potent vasopressor, to be given IV.

9. The rate of administration of the IV fluid containing norepinephrine is _______.
   a. maintained at the prescribed rate of infusion
   b. adjusted according to the patient's blood pressure
   c. given at a rate not to exceed five drops per minute
   d. discontinued when his blood pressure is 100 systolic
10. Mr. Alden's blood pressure should be monitored every _______.
    a. 3 to 5 minutes b. 15 to 30 minutes c. hour d. 3 to 4 hours
11. If intravenous fluid containing norepinephrine extravasates into subcutaneous tissue surrounding the needle site, _______.
    a. the IV is closely watched for further extravasation
    b. another IV line is immediately established and the IV containing norepinephrine is discontinued
12. While Mr. Alden is receiving the IV containing norepinephrine, he is _______.
    a. observed every 15 minutes
    b. placed in a semi-Fowlers position
    c. given a CNS depressant to lessen anxiety
    d. never left unattended

III. FILL-IN AND ESSAY QUESTIONS

Read each question carefully and place your answer in the space provided.

1. The peripheral nervous system consists of which two divisions or parts?
   1. _______________
   2. _______________
2. Another term or name for adrenergic drugs is
   ____
3. Adrenergic nerve fibers have either _______ or _______ receptors.
4. Norepinephrine and dopamine are given only by the _______ route of administration.
5. Leakage of an intravenous solution into surrounding tissues is called _______.
6. The nursing diagnosis *potential for infection* might be used when the patient is receiving an adrenergic drug. What is the contributing factor (or cause) that may initiate an infection in these patients?
   ____
   ____
   ____

7

Adrenergic Blocking Drugs

The following questions are concerned with the contents of Chapter 7, **Adrenergic Blocking Drugs**.

I. TRUE OR FALSE

Read each statement carefully and place your answer in the space provided.

1. _______ Alpha-Adrenergic blocking drugs produce their greatest effect on Beta-receptors.
2. _______ If stimulation of alpha-receptors is blocked or interrupted, the result will be vasodilatation.
3. _______ Stimulation of beta-receptors of the heart results in an increase in the heart rate.
4. _______ Antiadrenergic drugs may be used in the treatment of certain cardiac dysrhythmias and hypertension.
5. _______ Labetalol (Normodyne) is used primarily for the treatment of glaucoma.

II. MULTIPLE CHOICE QUESTIONS

Circle the letter of the most appropriate answer.

1. Alpha-adrenergic drugs are used mainly for their _______.
   a. central vasoconstricting effect
   b. ability to dilate veins
   c. vasodilating effect on peripheral blood vessels
   d. effect on the brain and spinal cord
2. An alpha-adrenergic blocking drug may be used in the treatment of _______.
   a. hypotension
   b. hypertension due to pheochromocytoma
   c. strokes
   d. cardiac dysrhythmias
3. Beta-adrenergic blocking drugs are primarily used in the treatment of _______.
   a. hypertension
   b. peripheral vascular disease
   c. mitral stenosis
   d. strokes

Clinical Situation I

Mr. Bates has hypertension and his physician decides to prescribe a beta-adrenergic blocking agent.

4. Prior to giving Mr. Bates the first dose of his drug, the most important physical assessment performed by the nurse would be _______.
   a. weighing Mr. Bates
   b. obtaining blood for laboratory tests
   c. taking a past medical history
   d. taking the blood pressure and pulse on both arms

5. Mr. Bates complains of dizziness and his pulse is now 58 beats per minute and his blood pressure has significantly decreased. His next dose of the drug is now due. Your next step would be to __d__.
   a. give the next dose but contact the physician
   b. advise Mr. Bates to ambulate in order to raise his blood pressure
   c. ask Mr. Bates to notify you if the dizziness becomes worse
   d. withhold the next dose and contact the physician
6. After several days of therapy Mr. Bates experiences postural hypotension, which is __a__.
   a. a feeling of lightheadedness or dizziness when changing position
   b. hypotension occurring when the patient is lying down
   c. a marked change in the blood pressure
   d. a decrease in the blood pressure and pulse rate when sitting
7. When giving Mr. Bates his medication, the nurse should __a__.
   a. take his blood pressure before the drug is given
   b. take his blood pressure 10 minutes after the drug is given

Clinical Situation II

Mrs. Slominski developed a life-threatening cardiac dysrhythmia and is receiving IV propranolol (Inderal).

8. While receiving this drug Mrs. Slominski will require __a__.
   a. constant medical supervision, cardiac monitoring, and frequent monitoring of her blood pressure and respiratory rate
   b. monitoring of her heart rate every 1 to 2 hours
   c. a private room, an ECG every hour, mechanical ventilation
9. When an adrenergic drug is given for a life-threatening cardiac dysrhythmia, the patient is placed on __d__.
   a. daily ECGs
   b. intake and output measured every 24 hours
   c. daily weights
   d. a cardiac monitor

III. FILL-IN AND ESSAY QUESTIONS

Read each question carefully and place your answer in the space provided.

1. Briefly explain the instructions that may be given to a patient experiencing postural hypotension.

   move slowly from standing sitting or lying position

2. Briefly explain or describe how you would take the blood pressure during the first week a patient is receiving a beta-adrenergic blocking agent for hypertension.

   Assess BP prior to giving hypertensive drug both arms standing sitting lying

3. A patient is receiving an adrenergic drug for hypertension and the blood pressure is stabilized. (1) How often is the blood pressure monitored? (2) Describe how the blood pressure is taken.

   1. prior to administration of the hypertensive drug
   2. take it in the same arm and position each time

4. List any four points you would include in a teaching plan for the patient receiving a beta-adrenergic blocking agent for hypertension.

1. Do not stop taking medication without doctors permission

2. Take medication same time each day

3. Dont take OTC drugs without consulting physician

4. Notify physician if adverse drug reaction occur

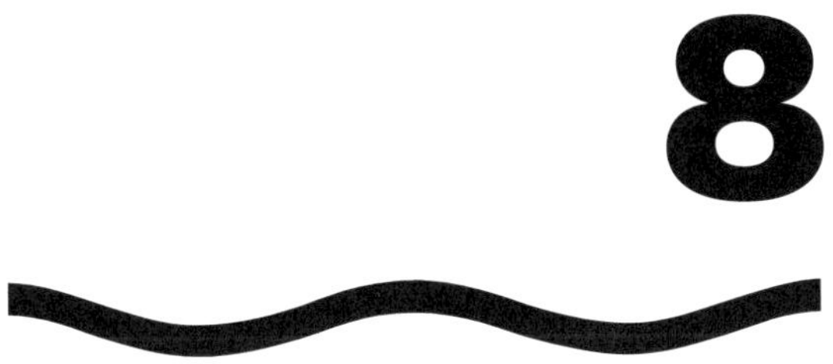

Cholinergic Drugs

The following questions are concerned with the contents of Chapter 8, **Cholinergic Drugs**.

I. TRUE OR FALSE

Read each statement carefully and place your answer in the space provided.

1. ______ Cholinergic drugs are also called parasympathomimetic drugs.
2. ______ The parasympathetic nervous system is part of the autonomic nervous system.
3. ______ Acetylcholinesterase is inactivated by acetylcholine.
4. ______ Generally, cholinergic drugs have limited use in medicine.
5. ______ Glaucoma may be treated with an ophthalmic cholinergic drug.
6. ______ A cholinergic drug may be given for urinary frequency.

II. MULTIPLE CHOICE QUESTIONS

Circle the letter of the most appropriate answer.

1. The parasympathetic nervous system is partly responsible for activities such as ______.
   1. slowing the heart rate
   2. movement in voluntary muscles
   3. the thought process
   4. eliminating body wastes

   a. 1, 2 b. 2, 3 c. 2, 4 d. 1, 4
2. The two neurohormones of the parasympathetic nervous system are ______.
   a. epinephrine, norepinephrine
   b. dopamine, ephedrine
   c. acetylcholine, acetylcholinesterase
3. Cholinergic drugs may act like the neurohormone ______.
   a. acetylcholine
   b. norepinephrine
4. When applied topically to the eye, a cholinergic drug such as pilocarpine will ______.
   a. dilate the pupil
   b. decrease the amount of redness in the eye
   c. increase intraocular pressure
   d. decrease intraocular pressure

Clinical Situation I

Mr. Stanford, age 43, has been diagnosed as having glaucoma.

5. For initial therapy, the physician orders pilocarpine eye drops. One adverse reaction that may occur with the use of this drug is ______.
   a. a temporary loss of visual acuity
   b. urinary retention
   c. dry mouth
   d. muscle weakness

6. Prior to instilling the eye drops, the nurse must check the label of the bottle to see if the drug is ______.
   a. for topical use
   b. sterile
   c. for ophthalmic use
   d. for glaucoma
7. Unless the physician orders otherwise, eye drops are instilled in the ______.
   a. outer corner (canthus) of the eye
   b. lower conjunctival sac
   c. upper conjunctival sac
   d. inner corner (canthus) of the eye
8. The hand holding the eye dropper is supported against the patient's ______.
   a. opposite cheek
   b. nose
   c. lower jaw
   d. forehead
9. The physician now allows Mr. Stanford to self-administer his eye drops and they are to be left at the bedside. The nurse ______.
   a. need not check Mr. Stanford, since a nurse is not giving the drug
   b. must check Mr. Stanford to be sure the medication is used properly and at the right time
10. Mr. Stanford's physician now prescribed a pilocarpine ocular system. This system is normally changed every ______.
    a. 4 hours   b. day   c. 7 days   d. month

Clinical Situation II

Ms. Martin has been diagnosed as having myasthenia gravis and is started on drug therapy with ambenonium (Mytelase).

11. During early drug therapy it will be important for the nurse to assess Ms. Martin for ______.
    a. the effects of the drug on her cardiovascular system
    b. muscle contractures
    c. dilatation of the pupils of her eyes
    d. her response to the drug
12. Assessment of Ms. Martin is important since the dose of the prescribed drug ______.
    a. usually must be increased every 4 hours
    b. frequently is increased or decreased early in therapy
    c. must be maintained at a certain level
    d. cannot be changed
13. The dose of a cholinergic drug for myasthenia gravis may be difficult to regulate and signs of overdose may occur. The signs of drug overdose include ______.
    a. muscle rigidity, clenching of the jaw
    b. muscle weakness, abdominal tenderness
    c. drop in blood pressure, diarrhea
    d. headache, double vision
14. Ms. Martin may also experience signs of drug underdose which may include ______.
    a. cardiac dysrhythmias, abdominal rigidity
    b. rapid fatigability of muscles, drooping of the eyelids
    c. salivation, clenching of the jaw
    d. anorexia, dyspnea
15. If drug overdose should occur, an antidote may be given. Which one of the following may be used as an antidote? ______
    a. morphine   b. pilocarpine   c. atropine   d. phenobarbital

III. FILL-IN AND ESSAY QUESTIONS

Read each of the following questions carefully and place your answer in the space provided.

1. Briefly describe how collected secretions due to insertion of the pilocarpine ocular system may be removed from the eye.

____

____

____

____

2. Briefly explain why the pilocarpine ocular system is best inserted at bedtime rather than during daytime hours.

Because their will be a temporary loss of visual acuity

3. Why is the nursing diagnosis *high risk for injury* applicable to the patient receiving an ophthalmic cholinergic preparation for the management of glaucoma?

The medication may cause ↓ of visual acuity that will make the pt prone to falls or injury.

9

Cholinergic Blocking Drugs

The following questions are concerned with the contents of Chapter 9, **Cholinergic Blocking Drugs**.

I. TRUE OR FALSE

Read each statement carefully and place your answer in the space provided.

1. ______ Cholinergic blocking drugs are also called anticholinergics.
2. ______ This group of drugs has an effect on the somatic part of the nervous system.
3. ______ Cholinergic blocking drugs may affect many organs and structures.
4. ______ Cholinergic blocking drugs increase gastric secretions.
5. ______ Cholinergic blocking drugs increase the heart rate.
6. ______ Responses to a cholinergic blocking drug may vary, depending on the drug and the dose used.
7. ______ The administration of a cholinergic blocking agent may result in frequent urination.
8. ______ Elderly patients usually tolerate these drugs very well, even when high doses are given.

II. MULTIPLE CHOICE QUESTIONS

Circle the letter of the most appropriate answer.

1. Cholinergic blocking drugs ______.
   a. inhibit the activity of acetylcholine
   b. enhance the effect of norepinephrine
   c. inhibit the activity of epinephrine
   d. enhance the effect of acetylcholine
2. Cholinergic blocking drugs are capable of ______.
   a. enhancing the effect of cholinergic drugs
   b. reversing the action of cholinergic drugs
3. A common adverse reaction of the cholinergic blocking drugs is ______.
   a. constriction of the pupil
   b. urinary frequency
   c. dryness of the mouth
   d. diarrhea
4. A cholinergic blocking drug such as atropine may be given before surgery to ______.
   a. inhibit the action of anesthesia
   b. reduce secretions of the upper respiratory tract
   c. inhibit the action of a preoperative narcotic
   d. increase gastric motility

5. Because of the effect of cholinergic blocking drugs on intestinal motility, patients taking these drugs for a long period of time may develop ______.
   a. gastric irritation due to an increase in gastric secretions
   b. diarrhea
   c. heartburn
   d. constipation
6. Administration of these drugs to elderly patients during the hot summer months may result in ______.
   a. an increase in sweating
   b. heat prostration
   c. a decrease in the heart rate
   d. intolerance to air conditioning
7. Cholinergic blocking drugs are contraindicated or used with caution in patients with ______.
   1. glaucoma
   2. a peptic ulcer
   3. an enlarged prostate
   4. diarrhea

   a. 1, 2 b. 1, 3 c. 2, 3 d. 2, 4
8. Atropine may be administered for ______.
   a. severe tachycardia
   b. third-degree heart block
   c. angina
9. When the patient is given atropine for the cardiac problem answered in question 8, he or she should be ______.
   a. placed on a cardiac monitor
   b. transferred to a private room
   c. placed in a supine position
   d. started on intravenous fluids
10. Patients with photophobia resulting from administration of a cholinergic blocking drug are usually more comfortable ______.
    a. in a cool room
    b. lying in bed
    c. in a semidarkened room
    d. in a brightly lit area

Clinical Situation

Mr. Baker has a peptic ulcer. He is currently being treated with the cholinergic blocking drug clidinium (Quarzan).

11. Mr. Baker complains of a dry mouth. Knowing the adverse reactions associated with these drugs, the nurse should ______.
    a. consider this to be unusual and contact the physician
    b. encourage Mr. Baker to take frequent sips of water
    c. give Mr. Baker salt-water mouth rinses
12. Although any patient complaint could be drug related, which of the following statements made by Mr. Baker are known to be the more common adverse reactions of a cholinergic blocking drug? ______
    1. "I haven't moved my bowels in several days."
    2. "I seem to be more nervous."
    3. "I have trouble reading the paper."
    4. "I don't enjoy watching television because the light bothers my eyes."
    5. "My legs hurt when I get out of bed."

    a. 1, 2, 4 b. 1, 3, 5 c. 1, 3, 4 d. 2, 4, 5
13. Mr. Baker's ulcer has begun to bleed and he is scheduled for surgery. Part of his preoperative medication is the cholinergic blocking agent glycopyrrolate (Robinul). After giving the drug, what information or instructions should be given to the patient? ______
    a. A severe dry mouth will occur; this is normal.
    b. You can remain out of bed until you get sleepy.
    c. In about one-half hour you should go to the bathroom and urinate.

III. FILL-IN AND ESSAY QUESTIONS

Read each question carefully and place your answer in the space provided.

1. Mydriasis may be defined as ______________________________.

2. Cycloplegia may be defined as ______________________________.

3. List or describe three daily assessments made when the patient is given a cholinergic blocking drug.

   1. assess vitial signs
   2. adverse drug reactions
   3. evaluate patients symptoms & complaints

4. Briefly explain why it is extremely important that a preoperative medication containing a cholinergic blocking drug be given at the prescribed time.

   the drug must be allowed to produce its greatest effect on the upper & lower respiratory system

5. Mr. Ward will be taking a cholinergic blocking drug following discharge from the hospital. The nurse first describes to him some of the adverse reactions that he might experience and may need to tolerate, and then suggests ways to lessen their intensity. Briefly explain what can be given to Mr. Ward for the following adverse reactions.

   Photophobia. ______

   Dry mouth. ______

   Constipation. ______

   Heat prostration. ______

   Drowsiness. ______

10

The Narcotic Analgesics and the Narcotic Antagonists

The following questions are concerned with the contents of Chapter 10, **The Narcotic Analgesics and the Narcotic Antagonists**.

I. TRUE OR FALSE

Read each statement carefully and place your answer in the space provided.

1. _______ Narcotics obtained from raw opium are synthetic narcotics.
2. _______ Morphine is a synthetic narcotic.
3. _______ Brompton's mixture is a mixture of an oral narcotic and another drug or drugs.
4. _______ How a narcotic relieves pain is not well understood.
5. _______ Administration of a narcotic analgesic results in the release of endorphins.
6. _______ Narcotics affect many organs and structures of the body.
7. _______ Morphine has a lesser miotic effect than codeine.
8. _______ Synthetic narcotics do not affect the respiratory center.
9. _______ Codeine may be used as an antitussive.
10. _______ A narcotic antagonist blocks the activity of narcotics, particularly their respiratory depressant effects.

II. MULTIPLE CHOICE QUESTIONS

Circle the letter of the most appropriate answer.

1. Brompton's mixture is used for _______.
   a. mild-to-moderate chronic pain
   b. chronic, severe pain
   c. the management of chronic arthritic diseases
   d. reversing the effects of morphine
2. If a narcotic has agonist properties, it is capable of _______.
   a. occupying the same opiate receptors as do enkephalins and endorphins
   b. destroying endorphins and enkephalins

3. Administration of a narcotic analgesic _______.
   a. lowers the pain threshold
   b. alters pain reception while lowering the pain threshold
   c. changes endorphins to enkephalins
   d. elevates the pain threshold and alters the perception of pain
4. Which of the following changes in the eye may be seen after the administration of morphine? _______
   a. mydriasis b. miosis c. myopia
5. What is the effect of morphine on respiration? _______
   a. The rate and depth is decreased.
   b. The rate is increased.
   c. The depth is decreased.
6. Morphine depresses the cough reflex. This is called an _______ effect.
   a. antireflex b. antiemetic c. antitussive d. antimedullary
7. Morphine _______.
   a. slows peristalsis in the stomach, duodenum, and small and large intestines
   b. increases the emptying time of the stomach
   c. increases gastric secretions
   d. increases intestinal peristalsis
8. The patient receiving morphine may experience nausea and vomiting because this drug _______.
   a. has antiemetic properties
   b. depresses the chemoreceptor trigger zone (CTZ)
   c. stimulates the pituitary gland
   d. stimulates the CTZ
9. Methadone may be given for pain but it is also used _______.
   a. when the patient is allergic to morphine
   b. in the detoxification and maintenance treatment of narcotic addiction
   c. to induce emesis following poison ingestion
   d. to stimulate respirations following anesthesia
10. One of the major hazards of narcotic administration is _______.
    a. pinpoint pupils
    b. respiratory depression
    c. lightheadedness
    d. euphoria
11. Patient-controlled analgesia _______.
    a. allows patients to administer their own analgesic
    b. appears to increase the need for narcotics in those with mild-to-moderate pain
    c. is only effective when oral narcotic analgesics are ordered
    d. decreases the time interval between doses of the narcotic
12. Narcotic antagonists are _______.
    a. used with narcotics to enhance the narcotic effect
    b. drugs capable of reversing the effects of narcotics
13. Which narcotic antagonist is used in the treatment of those formerly dependent on opioids? _______
    a. naltrexone b. naloxone
14. When administering naloxone it is important to _______.
    a. keep the patient's pulse rate below 100/minute
    b. restrain the patient
    c. keep the patient's respiratory rate below 16/minute
    d. maintain a patent airway

Clinical Situation

Mr. Dean, age 52, is receiving a narcotic for pain following surgery on his gallbladder.

15. Mr. Dean is experiencing pain. Prior to giving a narcotic the nurse should _______.
    1. ask Mr. Dean why he has pain
    2. assess the type and location of the pain
    3. take Mr. Dean's blood pressure, pulse, and respiratory rate
    4. check with the physician for approval to give the drug

    a. 1, 2, 3 b. 2, 3 c. 2, 3, 4 d. 1, 3
16. A narcotic should not be given to Mr. Dean if his respiratory rate is _______.
    a. 9/minute b. 14/minute c. 18/minute d. 20/minute

17. Mr. Dean receives his narcotic by the intramuscular route. Following administration the nurse must check his _______.
   a. relief of pain in 10 minutes
   b. alertness in 15 minutes
   c. blood pressure, pulse, and respiratory rate in 15 to 30 minutes
   d. pupils in 20 minutes
18. After Mr. Dean receives a narcotic he should be assessed for relief of pain in approximately _______.
   a. 10 minutes
   b. 20 to 30 minutes
   c. 1 hour
   d. 3 hours
19. Mr. Dean's blood pressure has averaged 140/90 for the past 3 days. Today, before giving him a narcotic, his blood pressure is 104/70. At this time the nurse should _______.
   a. give the narcotic since his systolic pressure is over 100
   b. ask Mr. Dean to wait another hour
   c. give the narcotic but check his blood pressure in 30 minutes
   d. not give the narcotic and contact his physician immediately
20. Miosis, which may occur with narcotic administration, _______.
   a. results in photophobia
   b. decreases the ability of the patient to see in dim light
   c. usually is accompanied by a headache
   d. interferes with the ability of the eye to focus

III. FILL-IN AND ESSAY QUESTIONS

Read each of the following questions carefully and place your answer in the space provided.

1. In planning nursing care of the patient receiving a narcotic analgesic following surgery, certain tasks, such as coughing, deep breathing, and leg exercises, are best done when the narcotic is producing its greatest effect. If Mr. Arnold receives a narcotic at 8 AM, when is the best time to perform these tasks?

   ____

2. Narcotic dependence (addiction) can occur if these drugs are given over a period of time. Why is drug dependence morally and ethically acceptable in the terminally ill cancer patient?

   ____

   ____

   ____

   ____

3. What observations and assessments are made when the patient receives a narcotic for the control of severe diarrhea?

   ____

   ____

   ____

4. List any four points you would include in a teaching plan for the patient with a prescription for a narcotic.
   1. ______________________________

      ____
   2. ______________________________

      ____
   3. ______________________________

      ____
   4. ______________________________

      ____

253

5. Describe how you would feel if you were in severe pain, requested something for your pain, and the nurse didn't return with your medication for 45 minutes.

___

___

___

___

___

11

The Non-Narcotic Analgesics

The following questions are concerned with the contents of Chapter 11, **The Non-Narcotic Analgesics**.

I. TRUE OR FALSE

Read each statement carefully and place your answer in the space provided.

1. _______ The salicylates have antipyretic activity.
2. _______ All of the salicylates are similar in pharmacologic activity.
3. _______ Salicylates lower an elevated body temperature by constricting peripheral blood vessels.
4. _______ Aspirin prolongs the bleeding time by inhibiting the aggregation (clumping) of platelets.
5. _______ Acetaminophen has anti-inflammatory activity and therefore is useful in treating the inflammatory process of arthritis.
6. _______ The nonsteroidal anti-inflammatory agents have anti-inflammatory, antipyretic, and analgesic activity.
7. _______ Acetaminophen may be useful for those with an aspirin allergy.
8. _______ The use of salicylates must be avoided for at least 1 week prior to any type of major or minor surgery.
9. _______ The nonsteroidal anti-inflammatory agents are of little value in the treatment of most arthritic disorders.
10. _______ Nonsteroidal anti-inflammatory agents have few, if any, adverse reactions.

II. MULTIPLE CHOICE QUESTIONS

Circle the letter of the most appropriate answer.

1. It is thought that the anti-inflammatory action of the salicylates is due to _______.
   a. their ability to dilate capillaries
   b. a direct action in higher nerve centers
   c. an indirect action on spinal cord nerves
   d. the inhibition of prostaglandins
2. Aspirin prolongs the bleeding time by _______.
   a. interfering with the manufacture of prothrombin
   b. inhibiting the aggregation of platelets
   c. a direct action on the liver
   d. increasing the manufacture of platelets
3. Acetaminophen has _______.
   a. analgesic and antipyretic activity
   b. analgesic activity only
   c. analgesic, antipyretic, and anti-inflammatory activity

4. The salicylates may be used in the treatment of inflammatory conditions such as _______.
   1. osteoarthritis
   2. mitral stenosis
   3. rheumatoid arthritis
   4. myocardial ischemia
   5. rheumatic fever

   a. 1, 4, 5 b. 1, 3, 5 c. 2, 3, 4 d. all of these
5. Salicylism may occur with salicylate overdose. Signs of mild salicylism include _______.
   a. nausea, vomiting, constipation
   b. insomnia, anxiety, headache
   c. dizziness, tinnitus, difficulty in hearing
   d. mental confusion, dyspnea, heartburn
6. Which of the following occurs with prolonged salicylate use? _______
   a. an increase in the ability of the blood to clot
   b. an increase in the number of platelets manufactured by the body
   c. loss of blood through the gastrointestinal (GI) tract
   d. a decrease in the number of white blood cells
7. Salicylates are contraindicated in those with _______.
   a. rheumatic fever with mitral stenosis
   b. a recent myocardial infarction
   c. blood dyscrasias, GI bleeding
   d. constipation
8. A salicylate should not be given, or given with great caution, to patients _______.
   1. with a bleeding peptic ulcer
   2. receiving anticoagulant therapy
   3. with a blood dyscrasia
   4. receiving an antineoplastic drug

   a. 1 only b. 1, 3, 4 c. 2, 3 d. all of these
9. Salicylates, especially aspirin, may be responsible for the development of _______.
   a. Reye's syndrome in children with chicken pox or influenza
   b. liver disorders
   c. intestinal polyps
   d. pancreatitis in adults
10. Adverse reactions associated with the use of acetaminophen usually occur _______.
    a. in those with inflammatory conditions
    b. with chronic use or when exceeding the recommended dosage
    c. when the drug is taken with an antacid
    d. if the patient is taking anticoagulants
11. Gastrointestinal reactions can occur with the use of the nonsteroidal anti-inflammatory drugs, especially in those _______.
    a. with rheumatoid arthritis
    b. with viral infections
    c. with a history of constipation
    d. prone to upper GI disorders

III. FILL-IN AND ESSAY QUESTIONS

Read each of the following questions carefully and place your answer in the space provided.

1. If the patient is given an oral salicylate for an elevated temperature, how soon after the drug is given should the temperature be checked?

   ____

2. Briefly describe the nursing assessments performed before the patient is started on therapy with a salicylate or nonsteroidal anti-inflammatory drug for an arthritic disorder.

   ____

   ____

   ____

   ____

   ____

3. List any four nursing diagnoses that may apply to the patient receiving a non-narcotic analgesic.

   1. ______________________________

      ____

   2. ______________________________

      ____

3. ______________________________

____

4. ______________________________

____

4. List any four points you would include in a teaching plan for the patient taking a non-narcotic analgesic.

1. ______________________________

____

2. ______________________________

____

3. ______________________________

____

4. ______________________________

____

12

Sedatives and Hypnotics

The following questions are concerned with the contents of Chapter 12, **Sedatives and Hypnotics**.

I. TRUE OR FALSE

Read each statement carefully and place your answer in the space provided.

1. _______ Hypnotics are given at night.
2. _______ Only the barbiturates are capable of producing central nervous system (CNS) depression.
3. _______ The rapid eye movement (REM) stage is the dreaming stage of sleep.
4. _______ Prior to administering a hypnotic it is important to know if the patient is comfortable and ready for sleep.
5. _______ Parenteral injection of a barbiturate in or near a peripheral nerve may result in permanent nerve damage.
6. _______ Hypnotics may be left at the bedside for the patient to take at a later hour.
7. _______ Excessive drowsiness or a headache may occur the morning after a hypnotic is given.
8. _______ Intramuscular injection of paraldehyde causes little or no discomfort.
9. _______ Drug dependency may develop with prolonged use of these drugs.
10. _______ A patient teaching plan should include a warning not to increase the dose of these drugs unless advised to do so by a physician.

II. MULTIPLE CHOICE QUESTIONS

Circle the letter of the most appropriate answer.

1. Over a period of time, sleep induced by the barbiturates _______.
   a. deprives an individual of the dreaming phase of sleep
   b. increases the respiratory rate during sleep
   c. increases the heart rate during sleep
   d. prolongs the REM stage of sleep
2. If an individual is deprived of the REM stage of sleep for a period of time, _______.
   a. sleep never lasts for more than 2 hours
   b. nightmares may occur
   c. anorexia becomes a problem
   d. a psychosis can develop
3. Barbiturates and nonbarbiturates are detoxified by the _______.
   a. spleen b. kidneys c. liver d. gastrointestinal tract

4. Sedatives are used chiefly in the treatment of _______.
   a. insomnia
   b. hypochondriasis
   c. anxiety and apprehension
   d. mental disorders

Clinical Situation

Mrs. Morris, age 53, is admitted for diagnostic tests. Her blood pressure, pulse, and respiratory rate data base are 150/82, 78, and 18, respectively. She had a breast biopsy this morning and will be discharged from the hospital tomorrow and readmitted in 1 week for a mastectomy.

5. Mrs. Norris tells you she has an arthritic condition and the pain keeps her awake at night. Will a barbiturate help relieve Mrs. Morris' pain? _______
   a. Yes, since these drugs have analgesic activity.
   b. No, because these drugs do not have analgesic activity.
6. Mrs. Morris received a narcotic analgesic at 9:45 PM and asks for her "sleeping pill" at 10 PM. Your decision is _______.
   a. not to give a hypnotic
   b. to give a hypnotic
7. The decision made in question 6 is based on the fact that _______.
   a. narcotics and barbiturates are both CNS depressants
   b. barbiturates do not depress the CNS
8. (If you selected *answer a* as the answer in question 7, answer this question and skip question 9. If you selected *answer b* as the answer in question 7, skip this question and answer question 9.) The reason *answer a* in question 7 is correct is that _______.
   a. two CNS depressant drugs given at the same time cancel the activity of both drugs
   b. severe respiratory depression may occur when two CNS depressant drugs are given
9. The reason *answer b* in question 7 is correct is that _______.
   a. only narcotics are true CNS depressants
   b. barbiturates do not affect the respiratory center
10. How long after a hypnotic is given is the patient assessed for drug effectiveness? _______
    a. 15 minutes b. 30 minutes c. 1 to 2 hours

III. FILL-IN AND ESSAY QUESTIONS

Read each of the following questions carefully and place your answer in the space provided.

1. Briefly define the following terms.

   Sedative. ____

   ____

   Hypnotic. ____

   ____

   Soporific. ____

   ____

2. Prior to the administration of a hypnotic, the nurse must assess the patient's needs. State three patient needs that may be identified prior to the administration of a hypnotic.

   1. ____
   2. ____
   3. ____

3. Briefly describe two nursing tasks related to patient safety that should be performed after the patient has received a hypnotic.

   1. ____

   ____

2. ____

____

4. Briefly state at least three areas or topics covered when developing a teaching plan for the patient prescribed a barbiturate or nonbarbiturate hypnotic.

1. ____

____

2. ____

____

3. ____

____

13

Substance Abuse

The following questions are concerned with the contents of Chapter 13, **Substance Abuse**.

I. TRUE OR FALSE

Read each statement carefully and place your answer in the space provided.

1. _______ When an individual is psychologically or physically dependent on a drug, there is a craving to use the drug repeatedly.
2. _______ Symptoms of the abstinence syndrome may vary.
3. _______ Heroin is obtained from codeine.
4. _______ Heroin is the strongest and most addicting of the opiates.
5. _______ A child born of a mother addicted to heroin is rarely addicted to heroin.
6. _______ Marijuana is classed as a CNS (central nervous system) stimulant.
7. _______ Although variable, the effects of marijuana usually last 2 to 4 hours.
8. _______ Mescaline and peyote produce effects similar to those of heroin.
9. _______ PCP is a hallucinogen.
10. _______ The amphetamines are adrenergic drugs.
11. _______ Tranquilizers are rarely abused.
12. _______ Alcohol abuse is a major problem in the United States.

II. MULTIPLE CHOICE QUESTIONS

Circle the letter of the most appropriate answer.

1. Symptoms of drug withdrawal are also called the _______ syndrome.
   a. physical b. dependency c. abstinence d. behavioral
2. Which of the following criteria apply to drug addiction? _______
   1. a compulsive desire to use a drug or chemical
   2. use of the drug affects only the individual
   3. a tendency to increase the dose
   4. a strong tendency to return to the drug after withdrawal
   5. no severe physical reactions when the drug is withdrawn

   a. 1, 2, 3 b. 1, 3, 4 c. 2, 4, 5 d. all of these
3. Which of the following criteria apply to drug habituation? _______
   1. use of the drug on an occasional basis
   2. little or no tendency to increase the dose
   3. no physical dependence
   4. psychological dependence

   a. 1, 2 b. 2, 3 c. 1, 4 d. 2, 4
4. Physical addiction to heroin _______.
   a. occurs rapidly
   b. is easy to cure
   c. is not detrimental to society
   d. occurs after months of use

5. Mrs. Bender has metastatic cancer and is terminally ill. She has been receiving a narcotic for 3 months and is now addicted to the drug. If her narcotic analgesic is not given as ordered and on time, _____.
   a. a larger dose will be required when the next dose is due
   b. a smaller dose should be given the next time the dose is due
   c. symptoms of narcotic withdrawal may occur
6. Cocaine _______.
   a. depresses the CNS
   b. has little, if any, effect on the CNS
   c. stimulates the CNS
7. Cocaine use may result in _______.
   a. physical dependence
   b. psychological dependence
   c. physical and psychological dependence
8. Which of the following are signs of chronic marijuana use? _______
   a. apathy, memory difficulty, carelessness in personal hygiene
   b. increased mental ability, nervousness, weight loss
   c. weight gain, increased reflexes, increased desire to improve oneself
   d. lack of motivation, time missed from work, physical dependence
9. The use of LSD may result in _______.
   a. an increase in productivity
   b. pronounced physical changes
   c. increased learning ability
   d. flashbacks
10. The amphetamines are used medically as/in _______.
    a. local anesthetics, emetics
    b. anorexiants, CNS stimulants
    c. the treatment of Reye's syndrome
    d. the management of manic-depressive patients
11. Use of the amphetamines may produce _______.
    a. euphoria, alertness, sense of excitation
    b. calmness, visual images, restlessness
    c. sensory deprivation, incoherence, lassitude
    d. talkativeness, dizziness, increased appetite
12. The amphetamines _______.
    a. are not addicting
    b. have addiction potential
13. Chronic use of the barbiturates can result in _______.
    a. physical and psychological dependence, drug tolerance
    b. physical dependence only
    c. drug intolerance, psychological dependence
14. Physical addiction to tranquilizers appears to _______.
    a. be less serious than addiction to other drugs
    b. occur only when low doses are taken
    c. be a problem only in those with severe anxiety
    d. occur fairly rapidly
15. In the treatment of substance abuse, success often depends on the _______.
    a. type of treatment program
    b. type of drug abused
    c. individual's desire to become drug-free

III. FILL-IN AND ESSAY QUESTIONS

Read each of the following questions carefully and place your answer in the space provided.

1. Define the following terms.

   Substance abuse. ______________________________

   ____

   ____

   Compulsive substance abuse. ______________________________

   ____

   ____

   Physical dependency. ______________________________

   ____

   ____

Psychological dependency. ______________________________

____

____

2. List any six signs of heroin withdrawal.
   1. ______________________________
   2. ______________________________
   3. ______________________________
   4. ______________________________
   5. ______________________________
   6. ______________________________
3. List or describe any three dangers associated with cocaine use.
   1. ______________________________
   2. ______________________________
   3. ______________________________
4. List or describe at least three problems associated with alcohol abuse.
   1. ______________________________
   2. ______________________________
   3. ______________________________

IV. Discussion

1. Drug abuse is a growing and serious problem in this country. Nurses, by the nature of their profession, are dedicated to helping the sick and injured. Nurses as well as other members of the medical profession have a significant incidence of drug abuse, including alcohol. The topic of drug use and abuse belongs in every school of nursing and should be considered carefully in light of the consequences that may develop when legal or illegal drugs are abused. The following general topics may be used for discussion. Other topics may also be relevant.
   1. The dangers of legal and illegal substance use
   2. Will trying an illegal drug just once do any harm?
   3. The future of the professional nurse who abuses drugs
   4. The legal consequences of substance abuse
   5. The professional license—can it be lost when the nurse abuses drugs?
   6. Drinking and driving—can it ruin a career?

14

The Cardiotonics and Antiarrhythmic Drugs

The following questions are concerned with the contents of Chapter 14, **The Cardiotonics and Antiarrhythmic Drugs**.

I. TRUE OR FALSE

Read each statement carefully and place your answer in the space provided.

1. ______ The cardiotonics are sometimes called cardiac glycosides.
2. ______ A glycoside is a synthetic substance comprised of a salt and one or more other chemicals.
3. ______ An increase in the heart rate places an added strain on the muscle of the heart.
4. ______ Digitalis toxicity can be serious.
5. ______ Digitoxin has the most rapid onset of action.
6. ______ The cardiotonics are relatively safe drugs.
7. ______ The antiarrhythmic drugs have the same mode of action as the cardiotonics.
8. ______ Some cardiac dysrhythmias result from many stimuli present in the myocardium.
9. ______ Cardiac muscle has the attributes of both nerve and muscle.
10. ______ Some cardiac dysrhythmias are caused by the generation of an abnormal number of electrical impulses (or stimuli).

II. MULTIPLE CHOICE QUESTIONS

Circle the letter of the most appropriate answer.

1. The primary difference between the cardiotonics is their ______.
   a. use in the treatment of cardiac dysrhythmias
   b. color
   c. duration and speed of action
   d. ability to increase the heart rate
2. Cardiac output is the ______.
   a. amount of blood leaving the left ventricle during each myocardial contraction
   b. total amount of blood pumped by the heart in 1 hour
   c. amount of blood entering the right ventricle
   d. amount of blood leaving the right ventricle during each myocardial contraction

3. Cardiotonic drugs have positive inotropic action, which is a(n) ______.
   a. decrease in the cardiac rate
   b. decrease in cardiac output
   c. increase in the electrical activity of the heart
   d. increase in the force of myocardial contraction
4. Cardiotonic drugs also ______.
   1. depress the SA node
   2. slow the conduction of the electrical impulse to the AV node
   3. stimulate the AV node
   4. increase the conduction of impulses to the bundle of His

   a. 1, 2 b. 1, 4 c. 2, 3 d. 3, 4
5. Cardiotonic drugs may be used in the treatment of ______.
   a. cardiac arrest, ventricular fibrillation
   b. congestive heart failure, some atrial dysrhythmias
   c. heart block, bigeminy pulse
6. The term digitalis toxicity refers to ______.
   a. a hypersensitivity reaction
   b. failure of a cardiotonic to correct a dysrhythmia
   c. toxic drug effects due to the administration of a cardiotonic
   d. toxicity occurring when a cardiotonic is given with an antiarrhythmic drug
7. Which nursing task must be performed prior to the administration of each dose of a cardiotonic? ______
   a. inspecting the extremities for edema
   b. measuring the intake and output
   c. reviewing the most recent ECG
   d. counting the pulse for 60 seconds
8. A cardiotonic should be withheld and the physician notified if the pulse rate ______.
   a. ranges between 60 and 80 per minute
   b. is regular
   c. is 60 per minute or below
9. During digitalization, the patient is observed for signs of digitalis toxicity every ______.
   a. day b. 12 hours c. 2 to 4 hours d. 15 minutes
10. Digitalis toxicity ______.
   a. only occurs when an overdose is given
   b. can occur when normal doses are given
   c. rarely occurs
   d. is usually not serious

Clinical Situation

Mr. Reynolds, age 51, is admitted to the hospital with a possible myocardial infarction. He has developed a cardiac dysrhythmia and his physician orders an antiarrhythmic drug.

11. Some cardiac dysrhythmias are caused by ______.
   a. the generation of an abnormal number of electrical impulses
   b. too much cholesterol in the diet
   c. a decrease in the size of the heart
   d. an increase in blood flow to the heart
12. When a patient is receiving an antiarrhythmic drug, the nurse should ______.
   a. take an apical and radial pulse every 1 to 4 hours
   b. monitor the intake and output every hour
   c. monitor the blood pressure daily
13. Mr. Reynolds is given disopyramide (Norpace) and has been experiencing a dry mouth, which may need to be tolerated. To relieve his discomfort the nurse may ______.
   a. suggest he have his family bring in ice cream
   b. offer him frequent sips of cool water
   c. suggest he drink less water
   d. offer him coffee between meals
14. The physician is notified if Mr. Reynolds' pulse rate ______.
   a. is below 80
   b. is above 80
   c. does not remain between 60 and 70
   d. is above 120 or below 60 per minute
15. If Mr. Reynolds will be taking disopyramide at home, the physician may want him to ______.
   a. monitor his own pulse rate
   b. measure his own intake and output
   c. eat a diet high in cholesterol
   d. avoid all forms of exercise

III. FILL-IN AND ESSAY QUESTIONS

Read each of the following questions carefully and place your answer in the space provided.

1. Give any six signs of digitalis toxicity.
   1. ______
   2. ______
   3. ______
   4. ______
   5. ______
   6. ______
2. List or describe any five of the initial assessments that should be performed before therapy with a cardiotonic drug is started.
   1. ______
   2. ______
   3. ______
   4. ______
   5. ______
3. List or describe five points that may be included in the teaching plan for a patient taking a cardiotonic drug.
   1. ______
   2. ______
   3. ______
   4. ______
   5. ______
4. List or describe any five of the initial assessments that should be performed before therapy with an antiarrhythmic drug is started.
   1. ______
   2. ______
   3. ______
   4. ______
   5. ______

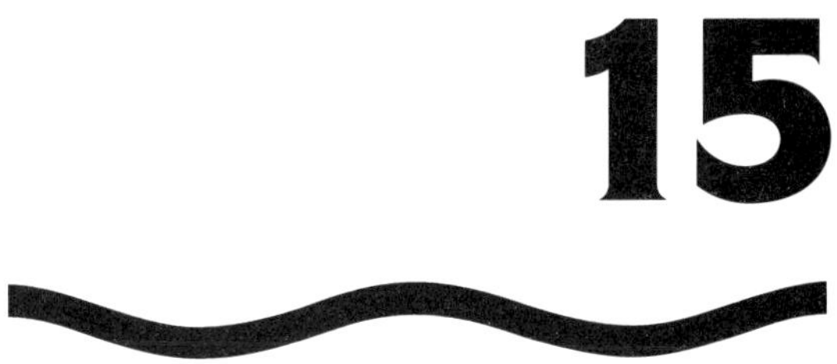

Anticoagulant and Thrombolytic Drugs

The following questions are concerned with the contents of Chapter 15, **Anticoagulant and Thrombolytic Drugs**.

I. TRUE OR FALSE

Read each statement carefully and place your answer in the space provided.

1. ______ Anticoagulants interfere with the clotting mechanism of the blood.
2. ______ The control value part of a prothrombin time is the patient's real prothrombin time.
3. ______ Clotting factor II is also called prothrombin.
4. ______ Heparin inhibits the formation of fibrin clots.
5. ______ Heparin can be given by the oral and subcutaneous routes.
6. ______ Heparin has no effect on clots that have already formed.
7. ______ Plasmin is an enzyme that breaks down fibrin.

II. MULTIPLE CHOICE QUESTIONS

Circle the letter of the most appropriate answer.

1. Anticoagulants are used to ______.
   a. shorten the prothrombin time
   b. prevent the formation of blood clots
   c. dissolve blood clots
   d. increase the number of platelets
2. Oral anticoagulants interfere with the ______.
   a. production of clotting factors by the reticuloendothelial system
   b. formation of clotting Factors I and II
   c. production of platelets by the bone marrow
   d. manufacture of vitamin-K-dependent clotting factors
3. In the stages of blood coagulation, injury results in the formation of ______.
   a. thromboplastin b. thrombokinin c. calcium
4. The principle adverse reaction associated with the use of oral anticoagulants is ______.
   a. loss of fibrinogen
   b. bleeding
   c. hypocalcemia
   d. liver damage

5. Heparin may be used to _______.
   1. dissolve pulmonary blood clots
   2. prevent venous thrombosis
   3. prevent a repeat cerebral thrombosis
   4. stop the activity of an oral anticoagulant
   a. 1, 2   b. 2, 3   c. 1, 3   d. 2, 4
6. Heparin is measured in _______.
   a. milligrams/liter
   b. units/milliliter
   c. milliunits/milliliter
7. Laboratory studies related to heparin therapy include a _______.
   a. prothrombin time, real prothrombin time
   b. CBC, sedimentation rate
   c. serum heparin studies
   d. PTT, whole blood clotting time
8. Intermittent IV heparin administration requires the use of an intermittent IV infusion set. If a lock flush solution is used, its purpose is to _______.
   a. remove the heparin from the IV needle
   b. clean the inner surface of the needle
   c. prevent small clots from obstructing the needle
   d. remove any small clots that have formed in the needle
9. If hemorrhage should occur during heparin administration, the physician may order _______.
   a. vitamin K therapy
   b. an oral anticoagulant
   c. protamine sulfate
10. Optimal therapeutic results of heparin therapy are obtained when the PTT is _______.
   a. 1-1/2 to 2-1/2 times the control value
   b. 2-1/2 to 3 times the control value
   c. between 6 and 10 minutes
11. Thrombolytic drugs are used to _______.
   a. lyse a thrombus
   b. prevent a thrombus from forming
   c. convert plasmin to plasminogen
   d. prevent the liver from manufacturing fibrin
12. The most frequent adverse reaction associated with the administration of thrombolytic drugs is _______.
   a. an increase in serum plasminogen
   b. a decrease in the PTT
   c. a decrease in the prothrombin time
   d. bleeding
13. Thrombolytic drugs are best given _______.
   a. when the prothrombin time is within normal limits
   b. within 6 hours after formation of a thrombus
   c. by the intramuscular route
   d. when the PTT is 3 to 3-1/2 times normal

Clinical Situation

Mr. Klein has had a myocardial infarction due to a coronary thrombosis. His physician orders an oral anticoagulant.

14. Prior to administering the first dose of the oral anticoagulant to Mr. Klein, _______.
   a. heparin must be given
   b. blood for a serum potassium level is drawn
   c. oral calcium must be given
   d. blood must be drawn for a baseline prothrombin time
15. Optimum results of oral anticoagulant therapy are obtained when the prothrombin time is _______.
   a. over 14 seconds
   b. 1-1/2 times the control value
   c. 1-1/2 to 2-1/2 times the control value
   d. under 25 seconds
16. If bleeding should occur during oral anticoagulant therapy, the physician may order _______.
   a. protamine sulfate
   b. vitamin K_1 (phytonadione)
   c. oral potassium supplements
   d. heparin
17. After two weeks of oral anticoagulant therapy, Mr. Klein's prothrombin time is 56 seconds and the control value is 13 seconds. This is _______.
   a. within normal limits
   b. low
   c. high
18. Mr. Klein develops an infection and is receiving an intramuscular antibiotic. Since he is on anticoagulant therapy, _______.
   a. prolonged pressure is applied to the needle site following each injection
   b. Mr. Klein is observed for signs that his prothrombin time is decreasing
   c. it will be necessary to double the dose of the anticoagulant

III. FILL-IN AND ESSAY QUESTIONS

Read each of the following questions carefully and place your answer in the space provided.

1. List any four areas that are checked for signs of bleeding when a patient is receiving an anticoagulant.

    1. emesis basin - vomitus
    2. oral & mucous membrane, skin
    3. stool, bed pan
    4. urine

2. List any five points you would include in a teaching plan for the patient taking an oral anticoagulant when at home.

    1. Use soft tooth brush.
    2. Follow the dosage schedule as prescribe by physician
    3. Take the drug at the same time each day
    4. If evidence of bleeding occurs, stop the next dose & call the doctor
    5. Do not take or discontinue the medication unless advise by the doctor

16

Antianginal Agents and Peripheral Vasodilating Drugs

The following questions are concerned with the contents of Chapter 16, **Antianginal Agents and Peripheral Vasodilating Drugs**.

I. TRUE OR FALSE

Read each statement carefully and place your answer in the space provided.

1. _______ Vasodilatation increases blood flow to an area.
2. _______ A peripheral vasodilator may be used in the treatment of peripheral vascular disorders.
3. _______ Calcium channel blockers are used primarily in the treatment of sustained hypotension.
4. _______ The nitrates have a direct relaxing effect on the smooth muscle layer of blood vessels, thereby producing vasoconstriction.
5. _______ Blanching of the skin is the chief adverse reaction seen with the peripheral vasodilators.
6. _______ Sublingual tablets are placed on the tongue.
7. _______ When ordered, sublingual nitroglycerin tablets may be left at the bedside.

II. MULTIPLE CHOICE QUESTIONS

Circle the letter of the most appropriate answer.

1. Peripheral vasodilators and the nitrates principally affect the _______.
   a. inner lining of blood vessels
   b. striated muscles of blood vessels
   c. smooth muscle layer of blood vessels
2. Calcium channel blockers _______.
   a. inhibit the movement of calcium ions across cell membranes
   b. increase the amount of calcium in the blood
   c. increase the movement of calcium across cell membranes
   d. decrease the activity of skeletal muscles

3. Administration of a peripheral vasodilator may result in ______.
   a. a decrease in the pulse rate
   b. an increase in the blood pressure
   c. moderate to severe diarrhea
   d. some degree of hypotension
4. When a patient receives a peripheral vasodilator for a peripheral vascular disorder, ______.
   a. improvement usually occurs slowly over a period of weeks
   b. ambulation is not allowed
   c. improvement is almost always rapid
   d. the legs must be kept elevated
5. Calcium channel blockers ______ the movement of calcium ions across cell membranes.
   a. enhance b. inhibit

Clinical Situation

Mrs. Trent is admitted to the hospital with chest pains. Her physician orders nitroglycerin as Nitro-Bid, which is an ointment applied topically, q8h. She is scheduled for several tests to determine the cause of her chest pain. She is allowed out of bed if she is not experiencing chest pain.

6. Before the drug is measured and applied, and after the ambulatory patient has rested for 10 to 15 minutes, the nurse ______.
   a. weighs the patient because the dose is based on weight
   b. checks the most recent laboratory tests for nitrate levels
   c. obtains the blood pressure and pulse rate
7. Nitro-Bid nitroglycerin ointment is applied to the skin by ______.
   a. rubbing it over an area of approximately 1 inch square
   b. spreading it in a thin uniform layer over a 6 × 6 inch area
8. The physician discontinues the use of topical nitroglycerin and orders nitroglycerin as a sublingual tablet. Normally, this form of nitroglycerin ______.
   a. is only given 3 to 4 times a day
   b. cannot be used more frequently than every half hour
   c. takes approximately one-half hour to relieve anginal pain
   d. may be used every 5 minutes until pain is relieved
9. After 1 week of therapy with sublingual nitroglycerin, the physician orders nitroglycerin in the form of a transdermal system. This form of the drug is applied ______.
   a. once a week b. every 4 hours c. once a day d. every 8 hours
10. Which of the following adverse reactions are commonly seen during initial therapy with the nitrates? ______
   a. hypertension b. headache c. bradycardia d. drowsiness

III. FILL-IN AND ESSAY QUESTIONS

Read each of the following questions carefully and place your answer in the space provided.

1. List any three initial physical assessments made prior to starting therapy with a peripheral vasodilator for a peripheral vascular disorder.
   1. ______
   2. ______
   3. ______
2. List any three characteristics of angina pain that should be noted during the initial assessment of the patient receiving an antianginal drug.
   1. ______
   2. ______
   3. ______

3. List any two points of information to include in a teaching plan for the patient using a transdermal nitroglycerin system.

1. apply the paste same time q day

2. Rotate sites each time you apply.

17

The Management of Body Fluids

The following questions are concerned with the contents of Chapter 17, **The Management of Body Fluids**.

I. TRUE OR FALSE

Read each statement carefully and place your answer in the space provided.

1. ______ The composition of body fluids remains relatively constant.
2. ______ Plasma must be typed and cross-matched prior to administration.
3. ______ Plasma may be given to the patient with severe burns.
4. ______ Intravenous fat emulsion is used to treat essential fatty acid deficiencies.
5. ______ 1000 mL of a 5% dextrose solution contains approximately 1500 calories.
6. ______ Sodium bicarbonate may be given for the treatment of respiratory alkalosis.
7. ______ Calcium is necessary for the clotting of blood.
8. ______ Magnesium plays an important role in the transmission of nerve impulses.
9. ______ Magnesium may be given by IV infusion.
10. ______ Oral sodium bicarbonate may be used to acidify the urine.

II. MULTIPLE CHOICE QUESTIONS

Circle the letter of the most appropriate answer.

1. Which of the following are contained in plasma? ______
   1. fats 2. electrolytes 3. sugar 4. proteins 5. bile pigments
   a. 1, 2, 4 b. 2, 3, 4 c. 2, 3, 5 d. all of these
2. Plasma protein fractions are used to treat ______.
   1. hypovolemic shock
   2. hepatic cirrhosis
   3. the diuretic syndrome
   4. the nephrotic syndrome
   a. all but 1 b. all but 2 c. all but 3 d. all but 4
3. Protein substrates are ______.
   a. small-molecule proteins
   b. amino acids
   c. fatty acids
   d. triglycerides
4. Plasma expanders may be used ______.
   a. until whole blood or plasma is available
   b. to decrease plasma volume
   c. in the treatment of hypervolemia

5. Fluid overload can occur with the administration of intravenous fluids. Signs of this condition include _______.
   1. decrease in the CVP
   2. behavioral changes
   3. distended neck veins
   4. decrease in blood pressure
   5. headache

   a. 1, 2, 4 b. 1, 3, 5 c. 2, 3, 5 d. 2, 4, 5
6. Calcium is necessary for the _______.
   1. clotting of blood
   2. digestion of food
   3. functioning of nerves and muscles
   4. manufacture of red blood cells

   a. 1, 3 b. 1, 4 c. 2, 3 d. 2 ,4
7. Magnesium is necessary for the _______.
   a. transmission of nerve impulses, activity of many enzyme reactions
   b. manufacture of blood plasma and red blood cells
   c. functioning of the parathyroid glands, cardiac function
   d. breakdown of starches, manufacture of hormones
8. Potassium may be given for hypokalemia, which may be seen in _______.
   1. severe vomiting
   2. diabetic acidosis
   3. marked diuresis
   4. severe malnutrition

   a. 1, 2 b. 2, 3 c. 3, 4 d. all of these
9. Sodium is essential for the _______.
   a. development of the bone matrix
   b. regulation of osmotic pressure in body cells
   c. digestion of food
   d. manufacture of plasma
10. Intravenous administration of calcium may result in _______.
    a. hypertension, diarrhea
    b. diuresis, potassium loss
    c. "heat waves," tingling
    d. headache, drowsiness
11. Prolonged or excessive use of sodium bicarbonate may result in _______.
    a. metabolic acidosis b. respiratory acidosis c. systemic alkalosis
12. Which of the following are signs of hypokalemia? _______
    a. leg cramps, decreased bowel sounds, muscle weakness
    b. hypertension, severe anxiety, poor skin turgor
    c. flaccid paralysis, tremors, weight gain
    d. bradycardia, cold clammy skin, diarrhea
13. Signs of hypernatremia include _______.
    a. weight gain, profuse diuresis, hypertension
    b. fever, hot dry skin, oliguria
    c. headache, cold clammy skin, hypotension
    d. bradycardia, constipation, anxiety

Clinical Situation

Mr. Edwards had major bowel surgery 4 weeks ago. Complications of his surgery include a draining fistula of the bowel and periodic episodes of vomiting, which required the insertion of a nasogastric tube.

14. What electrolyte imbalance might be occurring in Mr. Edwards? _______
    a. hypercalcemia
    b. hypoprothrombinemia
    c. hypokalemia
    d. hypernatremia
15. When serum electrolyte studies are done, it is noted that Mr. Edwards' serum sodium is low. His physician orders 2000 mL of 5% dextrose in normal saline. Normal saline is _______ sodium chloride.
    a. 0.2% b. 0.9% c. 0.45% d. 5%
16. Mr. Edwards will also require potassium. When potassium is given intravenously, it is _______.
    a. given undiluted
    b. given at a rapid rate
    c. always diluted before administration
17. When potassium is given IV it is not infused in less than _______.
    a. 3 to 4 hours b. 15 minutes c. 8 to 12 hours d. 24 hours
18. Following intravenous administration of potassium, oral potassium is ordered for Mr. Edwards. This drug is best given _______.
    a. on an empty stomach
    b. with food or immediately after meals

III. FILL-IN AND ESSAY QUESTIONS

Read each of the following questions carefully and place your answer in the space provided.

1. List at least three points or areas of patient instruction to accompany the prescription of a potassium salt.

   1. Tablets must not be crushed or chewed

   2. must be taken on a full stomach or after meals

   3. Must be administerd slowly po 10-20 min / IV over 4-6 hrs Max 40 mEq.

18

Diuretics and Antihypertensive Drugs

The following questions are concerned with the contents of Chapter 18, **Diuretics and Antihypertensive Drugs**.

I. TRUE OR FALSE

Read each statement carefully and place your answer in the space provided.

1. _______ A diuretic promotes the excretion of water and electrolytes.
2. _______ Carbonic anhydrase inhibitors are used in the treatment of decreased intraocular pressure.
3. _______ Loop diuretics are particularly useful when a greater diuretic effect is desired.
4. _______ Aldosterone is a hormone produced by the kidney.
5. _______ Adverse reactions are rare when a carbonic anhydrase inhibitor is used for short-term therapy.
6. _______ The patient should be weighed prior to the administration of the first dose of a diuretic for edema.
7. _______ Most cases of hypertension have a known cause.
8. _______ Weighing the patient at regular intervals is usually necessary if the patient is on a weight-reduction diet as part of the therapeutic regimen for hypertension.
9. _______ The blood pressure is monitored daily if the patient has severe hypertension.
10. _______ An antihypertensive drug is withheld if the blood pressure has decreased significantly since the last reading.

II. MULTIPLE CHOICE QUESTIONS

Circle the letter of the most appropriate answer.

1. Most diuretics act on the _______.
   a. glomerulus
   b. renal collecting system
   c. tubules of the kidney nephron
2. As the filtrate (fluid removed from the blood) passes through the proximal tubule, the loop of Henle, and the distal tubules, _______ of amino acids, glucose, some electrolytes, and water takes place.
   a. excretion
   b. electrolyte binding
   c. electrolyte dissociation
   d. selective reabsorption

3. Carbonic anhydrase produces free hydrogen ions which are then exchanged for _a_ ions in the kidney tubules.
   a. sodium b. potassium c. chloride d. calcium
4. Inhibition of the enzyme carbonic anhydrase results in the excretion of _a_ ions.
   a. sodium b. calcium c. magnesium d. carbonate
5. Loop diuretics _c_.
   a. enhance the reabsorption of sodium ions in the distal and proximal loops
   b. promote excretion of water by adding sodium ions to the filtrate in the glomerulus
   c. inhibit the reabsorption of sodium and chloride ions in the distal and proximal tubules and the loop of Henle
6. Osmotic diuretics increase the density of the filtrate in the _b_.
   a. loop of Henle b. glomerulus c. distal tubule d. proximal tubule
7. If a patient with acute glaucoma is receiving acetazolamide (Diamox), a carbonic anhydrase inhibitor, the nurse should _b_.
   a. monitor the blood pressure and pulse every 15 to 30 minutes
   b. check the patient's relief of eye pain q2h
   c. look for signs of decreased peripheral edema
   d. check the pupil in the unaffected eye for miosis
8. Many antihypertensive drugs lower the blood pressure by _b_.
   a. enhancing the retention of sodium in the kidney tubules
   b. dilating arterial blood vessels
   c. direct action on spinal cord nerves
   d. constricting venules
9. Early in therapy, some patients receiving an antihypertensive drug may experience _c_.
   a. acute hypertensive episodes
   b. difficulty urinating
   c. orthostatic and/or postural hypotension
   d. shortness of breath
10. Prior to each administration of an antihypertensive drug, the _d_.
   a. patient is weighed
   b. extremities are checked for edema
   c. apical-radial pulse is obtained
   d. blood pressure and pulse rate are obtained
11. The patient taking an antihypertensive drug is told not to use any nonprescription drug unless use has been approved by the physician. The reason for this is some nonprescription products _a_.
   a. may contain a drug capable of raising the blood pressure
   b. may contain an antihypertensive drug

Clinical Situation

Mr. Woods has been prescribed a thiazide diuretic because he has early and mild congestive heart failure.

12. The thiazide diuretics _a_.
   a. promote the reabsorption of sodium and chloride ions
   b. increase serum sodium levels
   c. inhibit the reabsorption of sodium and chloride ions
   d. promote the reabsorption of potassium ions
13. Administration of any diuretic may result in an electrolyte imbalance. Since Mr. Woods is receiving a thiazide diuretic, he is observed for signs of _b_, which is the most common electrolyte imbalance seen with the administration of most diuretics.
   a. hypernatremia
   b. hypokalemia
   c. metabolic alkalosis
   d. hyperkalemia
14. Because of a severe electrolyte loss, the physician discontinues the thiazide diuretic and orders the potassium-sparing diuretic spironolactone (Aldactone). This drug _c_.
   a. increases the excretion of potassium
   b. decreases the excretion of sodium ions
   c. will conserve potassium
15. After a period of time, the diuretic effect of a diuretic drug may be minimal, because most of the body's excess fluid has been removed. Mr. Wood should be told that _a_.
   a. therapy may be continued to prevent further accumulation of fluid
   b. therapy will be discontinued once his lungs are clear and the edema subsides

III. FILL-IN AND ESSAY QUESTIONS

Read each of the following questions carefully and place your answer in the space provided.

1. List any four assessments made when the patient with edema is receiving a diuretic.

   1. daily weight
   2. monitor intake & output
   3. vital signs q 1-4h
   4. Check areas of edema to evaluate the effectiveness of the drug

2. Mr. Wells has been prescribed a diuretic for peripheral edema. List or describe any four areas of information that may be included in the teaching plan for this patient.

   1. Do not stop the drug unless c̄ the advise of a physician
   2. Avoid alcohol and nonprescription drugs unless they has been approved by the physician.
   3. Take drug once a day early in the morning unless otherwise advise
   4. After a time diuretic results will be less.

3. Briefly explain why it is important to monitor the blood pressure of the patient receiving an antihypertensive drug.

   To evaluate the drug response
   Drug dosage may require adjustments
   drug may need to be discontinue or another
   drug added to the regimen

4. What advice can the nurse give to the patient experiencing postural hypotension during therapy with an antihypertensive drug?

   rise from a sitting or lying position
   slowly

19

Central Nervous System Stimulants

The following questions are concerned with the contents of Chapter 19, **Central Nervous System Stimulants**.

I. TRUE OR FALSE

Read each statement carefully and place your answer in the space provided.

1. _______ The amphetamines appear to act on the appetite center of the spinal cord.
2. _______ Caffeine stimulates all levels of the central nervous system.
3. _______ Long-term use of the amphetamines in the treatment of obesity is not recommended.
4. _______ Amphetamines can raise the blood pressure.
5. _______ Methylphenidate (Ritalin) is used in the treatment of respiratory depression.

II. MULTIPLE CHOICE QUESTIONS

Circle the letter of the most appropriate answer.

1. The analeptic doxapram (Dopram) stimulates the respiratory center, which is located in the _______.
   a. cerebellum
   b. medulla
   c. cerebrum
   d. thoracic section of the spinal cord
2. Doxapram may be used in the treatment of _______.
   1. drug-induced respiratory depression
   2. respiratory depression in chronic pulmonary disease
   3. congestive heart failure
   4. narcolepsy

   a. 1, 2 b. 1, 3 c. 2, 4 d. 3, 4
3. The amphetamines _______.
   a. are of little value in the treatment of narcolepsy
   b. are not true CNS stimulants
   c. have abuse and addiction potential
   d. have some CNS depressant effects
4. Nonprescription diet aids containing phenylpropanolamine have _______.
   a. actions similar to the analeptics
   b. great abuse and addiction potential
   c. use in the treatment of behavior disorders in children
   d. limited appetite-suppressing ability when compared with the anorexiants

5. Methylphenidate is used in the treatment of _______.
   1. exogenous obesity
   2. narcolepsy
   3. respiratory depression
   4. attention deficit disorders in children
   a. 1, 2 b. 2, 4 c. 1, 3 d. 1, 4
6. Overstimulation may occur with use of a CNS stimulant and result in _______.
   a. insomnia, tachycardia, nervousness
   b. dizziness, bradycardia, hypotension
   c. anxiety, hypotension, anorexia
   d. sleepiness, hypertension, vertigo
7. Following administration of a CNS stimulant for respiratory depression, the respiratory rate is monitored until the rate is _______.
   a. 10 or below b. normal c. less than 24 per minute
8. Initial assessment of the child with an attention deficit disorder should include _______.
   a. seeing if the child responds to physical stimuli
   b. a determination of the child's intelligence
   c. a summary of the behavior pattern
   d. removing all physical stimuli from the environment

III. FILL-IN AND ESSAY QUESTIONS

Read each question carefully and place your answer in the space provided.

1. Briefly list the initial assessments made prior to the administration of a CNS stimulant for respiratory depression.

____

____

____

20

Insulin and Oral Hypoglycemic Drugs

The following questions are concerned with the contents of Chapter 20, **Insulin and Oral Hypoglycemic Drugs**.

I. TRUE OR FALSE

Read each statement carefully and place your answer in the space provided.

1. _______ Insulin is a hormone manufactured by the beta cells of the pancreas.
2. _______ The onset of insulin occurs when this hormone first begins to act in the body.
3. _______ Insulin may be necessary for the more severe and complicated forms of Type II diabetes mellitus.
4. _______ Insulin is rarely necessary for Type I diabetes mellitus.
5. _______ On rare occasions, an individual may be allergic to insulin.
6. _______ Insulin injection sites are rotated.
7. _______ Hypoglycemia does not occur with the use of the oral hypoglycemic drugs.
8. _______ Anorexia, epigastric discomfort, and various neurologic symptoms are adverse reactions to the oral hypoglycemic drugs.
9. _______ A diabetic may require insulin *and* an oral hypoglycemic agent.
10. _______ The urine of the diabetic receiving an oral hypoglycemic drug need not be tested for glucose.

II. MULTIPLE CHOICE QUESTIONS

Circle the letter of the most appropriate answer.

Clinical Situation I

Mrs. White, age 41, is a newly diagnosed diabetic. Her physician has determined that it is necessary to begin treatment with insulin.

1. Insulin appears to activate a process that _______.
   a. moves glucose from smooth muscle to the bloodstream
   b. changes glucose into a starch
   c. removes glucose from the cells of striated muscle
   d. helps glucose enter the cells of striated muscle and adipose tissue

2. Mrs. White will receive regular insulin, which is a rapid-acting insulin that has an onset of action in approximately _______.
   a. 5 to 10 minutes
   b. 15 to 20 minutes
   c. 30 to 60 minutes
   d. 1 to 2 hours
3. Mrs. White is diagnosed as having Type I diabetes mellitus which is also known as _______.
   a. insulin-dependent diabetes mellitus
   b. maturity-onset diabetes mellitus
   c. diabetes mellitus of unknown origin
4. Mrs. White may develop hypoglycemia, which can occur when there is _______.
   a. too much insulin in the bloodstream in relation to available glucose
   b. too much glucose in the cells
   c. a decreased amount of insulin in the bloodstream in relation to available glucose
   d. an insufficient amount of glucose in the cells
5. Hypoglycemia can occur when the _______.
   1. patient eats too little food
   2. patient eats too much food
   3. insulin dose taken is greater than that prescribed
   4. insulin dose taken is smaller than that prescribed
   5. patient drastically increases physical activity
   6. patient drastically decreases physical activity

   a. 1, 3, 5 b. 2, 4, 6 c. 1, 2, 5 d. 2, 4, 6
6. When obtaining an initial history from Mrs. White, it is important to ask her _______.
   1. about the type and duration of symptoms she has experienced
   2. about her dietary habits
   3. if there is a family history of diabetes
   4. if she is allergic to insulin

   a. all but 1 b. all but 2 c. all but 3 d. all but 4
7. Mrs. White is receiving regular insulin, which is given _______.
   a. once a day, between 6 and 8 AM
   b. 15 to 30 minutes before a meal
   c. once a day at HS
   d. immediately after the noon meal
8. If Mrs. White should have a hypoglycemic reaction, she can only be given an oral fluid or substance to terminate this reaction when _______.
   a. the hypoglycemic reaction occurs at least 2 hours after she has received her insulin
   b. a physician has seen her having a hypoglycemic reaction
   c. her swallowing and gag reflexes are present
9. The urine of a hospitalized diabetic is checked for glucose and ketones _______.
   a. every morning before breakfast
   b. 4 times a day, before meals, and at HS
   c. 2 times a day, early morning, and at HS
   d. every 2 hours
10. Mrs. White's physician is notified if her urine is positive for ketones or the glucose is above _____.
   a. 1% b. 0.1% c. 0.25% d. 3%
11. Before discharge from the hospital, Mrs. White's insulin is changed to protamine zinc insulin. When insulin is combined with protamine, absorption from the injection site is _______ and the duration of action is _______.
   a. more rapid, prolonged
   b. slowed, prolonged
   c. slowed, decreased
   d. more rapid, decreased

Clinical Situation II

Mr. Otis, age 59, has been diagnosed as having Type II diabetes mellitus. His physician has prescribed an oral hypoglycemic agent.

12. Oral hypoglycemic agents appear to lower blood glucose by _______.
   a. stimulating beta cells of the pancreas to release insulin
   b. moving glucose from the bloodstream to the cells
   c. allowing insulin to enter body cells
   d. direct stimulation of the pancreatic duct
13. Oral hypoglycemic agents are only of value for those with Type II diabetes mellitus who _______.
   a. are age 50 and over
   b. have inactive alpha and beta pancreatic cells
   c. are allergic to insulin
   d. cannot be controlled by diet alone
14. An oral hypoglycemic agent is usually given _______.
   a. 30 minutes before each meal
   b. as a single daily dose or in divided doses

15. During initial therapy with an oral hypoglycemic agent, Mr. Otis should be observed for a hypoglycemic reaction _______.
   a. daily
   b. after meals
   c. 15 to 30 minutes after the drug is given
   d. every 2 to 4 hours
16. If Mr. Otis were to have a hypoglycemic reaction, it _______.
   a. will most likely occur 1 to 2 hours after a meal
   b. may be more intense than one seen with insulin administration
   c. may be less intense than one seen with insulin administration

III. FILL-IN AND ESSAY QUESTIONS

Read each of the following questions carefully and place your answer in the space provided.

1. The two major adverse reactions seen with the administration of insulin are ____________________ and ____________________.
2. Name any six signs and symptoms of hypoglycemia.
   1. ____________________
   2. ____________________
   3. ____________________
   4. ____________________
   5. ____________________
   6. ____________________
3. Name any six signs and symptoms of hyperglycemia.
   1. ____________________
   2. ____________________
   3. ____________________
   4. ____________________
   5. ____________________
   6. ____________________
4. Name any four preparations that may be used to terminate a hypoglycemic reaction.
   1. ____________________
   2. ____________________
   3. ____________________
   4. ____________________
5. List or describe any 10 points that may be included in a teaching plan for a newly diagnosed diabetic patient who will be self-administering insulin.
   1. ____________________
   2. ____________________
   3. ____________________
   4. ____________________

5. ____

____

6. ____

____

7. ____

____

8. ____

____

9. ____

____

10. ____

____

6. List any five points that are included in a teaching plan for a newly diagnosed diabetic patient who will be taking an oral hypoglycemic drug.

1. ____

____

2. ____

____

3. ____

____

4. ____

____

5. ____

____

21

The Sulfonamides

The following questions are concerned with the contents of Chapter 21, **The Sulfonamides**.

I. TRUE OR FALSE

Read each statement carefully and place your answer in the space provided.

1. __T__ Sulfonamides are mostly bacteriostatic.
2. __F__ Adverse reactions to the sulfonamides are rarely serious.
3. __T__ Crystalluria may be defined as crystals in the urine.
4. __T__ Sulfasalazine (Azulfidine) may be used for the management of ulcerative colitis.
5. __F__ Unless the physician orders otherwise, the sulfonamides are given with meals.

II. MULTIPLE CHOICE QUESTIONS

Circle the letter of the most appropriate answer.

1. The anti-infective ability of the sulfonamides is due to their ability to _______.
   a. encourage the formation of antibodies
   b. antagonize PABA, a substance that some bacteria need to multiply
   c. increase the number of white blood cells
2. The sulfonamides are used chiefly to _______.
   a. treat upper respiratory tract infections
   b. control bacterial growth in the small bowel
   c. treat generalized infections
   d. control urinary tract infections caused by certain bacteria
3. The Stevens-Johnson syndrome is an allergic reaction that may occur during administration of a sulfonamide. Signs of this reaction include _______.
   a. lesions on various areas of the body, fever, cough
   b. hypotension, tachycardia, diarrhea
   c. low body temperature, constipation, bradycardia
   d. convulsions, hair loss, drop in the white blood cell count
4. Another adverse reaction to the sulfonamides is crystalluria, which may be prevented by _______.
   a. keeping the urine output below normal
   b. increasing the fluid intake
   c. keeping the urine acidic
   d. eating foods high in purine
5. The most frequent adverse reaction of mafenide (Sulfamylon), a topical sulfonamide used in the treatment of severe burns, is _______.
   a. crystalluria
   b. proteinuria
   c. a burning sensation or pain
   d. edema
6. Unless the physician orders otherwise, sulfonamides are best given _______.
   a. with meals
   b. with cranberry juice
   c. with milk
   d. 1 hour before or 2 hours after meals

7. Patients receiving a sulfonamide preparation are encouraged to _______.
   a. decrease their fluid intake
   b. increase their fluid intake to 2000 mL or more per day
   c. ambulate frequently
   d. drink carbonated beverages
8. When a topical sulfonamide is used in the treatment of burns, the drug is applied to the burned areas _______.
   a. every 24 hours
   b. with a sterile gloved hand
   c. with cotton wads or balls
9. If the patient is diabetic and is receiving the oral hypoglycemic agent tolbutamide (Orinase) and a sulfonamide, he is watched closely for signs of _______.
   a. hypoglycemia b. hyperglycemia

III. FILL-IN AND ESSAY QUESTIONS

Read each of the following questions carefully and place your answer in the space provided.

1. List or describe any five areas or points to be included in a teaching plan for the patient taking a sulfonamide drug.
   1. Take the medication as prescribed
   2. maintain follow-up care to ensure the infection is controlled.
   3. Take drug on empty stomach either 1 hour before or 2 hour after eating
   4. Do not increase or decrease the time between doses unless directed by physician
   5. Prolonged exposure to sunlight may result in skin reaction

22

The Penicillins and the Cephalosporins

The following questions are concerned with the contents of Chapter 22, **The Penicillins and the Cephalosporins**.

I. TRUE OR FALSE

Read each statement carefully and place your answer in the space provided.

1. _______ Bacterial resistance rarely occurs with the use of penicillin.
2. _______ The penicillins may be bactericidal or bacteriostatic.
3. _______ Penicillin has value in the treatment of viral and fungal infections.
4. _______ The cephalosporins are structurally and chemically related to penicillin.
5. _______ When penicillin or a cephalosporin is given IM, there may be pain at the injection site.

II. MULTIPLE CHOICE QUESTIONS

Circle the letter of the most appropriate answer.

1. When a patient is allergic to penicillin, there is an increased possibility that he will also be allergic to _______.
   a. erythromycin
   b. the tetracyclines
   c. chloramphenicol
   d. the cephalosporins
2. If a patient is allergic to one penicillin, there is an increased possibility that he will be allergic to all of the penicillins. This is called _______.
   a. cross-resistance
   b. cross-sensitivity or cross-allergenicity
   c. a sensitive-resistant reaction
   d. relative resistance
3. The cephalosporins are usually _______.
   a. bactericidal b. bacteriostatic
4. The cephalosporins may be used during the preoperative, intraoperative, and postoperative period to prevent infections in those having surgery _______.
   a. that requires a general anesthetic
   b. that requires a local anesthetic or spinal anesthetic
   c. on a contaminated or potentially contaminated area
   d. on the lower extremities
5. The laboratory test performed to determine if a specific bacteria is sensitive to penicillin is a _______.
   a. penicillin resistance test
   b. sensitivity test
   c. CBC and differential
   d. culture

6. A problem associated with the use of penicillin as well as other antibiotics is superinfection, which is a(n) _______.
   a. viral infection affecting the respiratory system
   b. infection that occurred before the penicillin was given
   c. bacterial or fungal overgrowth of microorganisms not susceptible to penicillin
   d. infection due to protozoa

Clinical Situation

Mr. Patterson has developed a wound infection following abdominal surgery. After reviewing the results of culture and sensitivity tests, the physician prescribes penicillin.

7. Penicillin for Mr. Patterson may be ordered in _______.
   1. grains 2. milligrams 3. units 4. micrograms
   a. 1, 2 b. 2, 3 c. 1, 3 d. 2, 4
8. In order for penicillin to be effective, _______.
   a. adequate blood levels of the drug must be maintained
   b. it must be given with meals
   c. it must be given by the parenteral route
9. If Mr. Patterson should have a minor hypersensitivity reaction to penicillin, treatment may include _______.
   a. administration of an antihistamine
   b. administration of penicillinase
   c. steroid baths
   d. starting an IV containing epinephrine
10. Which of the following may indicate Mr. Patterson has developed a superinfection? _______
    1. sore mouth and throat
    2. itching around the anal area
    3. constipation
    4. edema of the extremities
    5. chills and fever
    a. 1, 4, 5 b. 2, 3, 4 c. 1, 2, 5 d. 3, 4, 5
11. Which one of the following may indicate Mr. Patterson is responding to penicillin therapy? A(n) _______.
    a. increase in his white blood cell count
    b. decrease in the amount of drainage from his surgical wound
    c. rise in his temperature
    d. decrease in his red blood cell count

III. FILL-IN AND ESSAY QUESTIONS

Read each of the following questions carefully and place your answer in the space provided.

1. Mr. Kelly is admitted to the hospital with a draining and infected leg ulcer and is to be started on a cephalosporin. List or describe the observations that should be made during the initial physical assessment of the leg ulcer that will provide baseline data for comparison during therapy with an antibiotic.

   ____

   ____

   ____

   ____

2. List any five points or areas that would be included in a teaching plan for the patient with an infection and prescribed penicillin for use on an out-patient basis.
   1. ______________________________
   2. ______________________________
   3. ______________________________
   4. ______________________________
   5. ______________________________

23

The Broad-Spectrum Antibiotics and Antifungal Drugs

The following questions are concerned with the contents of Chapter 23, **The Broad-Spectrum Antibiotics and Antifungal Drugs**.

I. TRUE OR FALSE

Read each statement carefully and place your answer in the space provided.

1. _______ Broad-spectrum antibiotics may be bactericidal or bacteriostatic.
2. _______ Sensitivity tests are usually not necessary when the use of broad-spectrum antibiotics is being considered for the control of an infection.
3. _______ Administration of chloramphenicol (Chloromycetin) can result in serious and sometimes fatal blood dyscrasias.
4. _______ There is a high incidence of serious adverse reactions associated with the oral administration of the erythromycins.
5. _______ A fungus is a colorless plant lacking chlorophyll.
6. _______ A fungal infection may also be called a mycotic infection.
7. _______ Antifungal drugs are also used for many types of bacterial infections.
8. _______ When applied topically, there are few adverse reactions associated with the use of an antifungal drug.

II. MULTIPLE CHOICE QUESTIONS

Circle the letter of the most appropriate answer.

1. Mr. Layne has a viral infection and his physician orders a broad-spectrum antibiotic. The rationale for use of an antibiotic for Mr. Layne is _______.
   a. this group of drugs is effective against most viruses
   b. a secondary bacterial infection may potentially occur
   c. all viral infections are accompanied by bacterial infections

2. Two antibiotics used prior to bowel surgery to reduce the number of bacteria normally present in the intestine are _______.
   a. clindamycin (Cleocin) and tetracycline
   b. chloramphenicol (Chloromycetin) and bacitracin
   c. amikacin (Amikin) and erythromycin
   d. kanamycin (Kantrex) and neomycin (Mycifradin)
3. Bacterial superinfections often occur in the _______.
   a. bowel
   b. liver
   c. pancreas
   d. kidneys
4. A photosensitivity reaction may be seen during use of the tetracyclines and is manifested by a(n) _______.
   a. aversion to bright light
   b. blue-brown pigmentation of the skin
   c. exaggerated sunburn reaction after brief exposure to sunlight
   d. increased wrinkling of the skin
5. Ototoxicity may occur with the use of some broad-spectrum antibiotics. Symptoms of this adverse reaction include _______.
   a. tinnitus, mild-to-severe hearing loss
   b. dizziness, difficulty swallowing
   c. dyspnea, nausea
   d. increased nasal discharge, vertigo
6. Nephrotoxicity may also occur with the use of some broad-spectrum antibiotics. Symptoms of this adverse reaction include _______.
   a. decreased BUN and serum creatinine
   b. oliguria, protein in the urine
   c. anuria, dysuria
   d. increased urinary output, decreased serum creatinine
7. Parenteral administration of amphotericin B (Fungizone IV), an antifungal agent, _______.
   a. rarely results in serious adverse reactions
   b. requires that the infusion be given in 2 or less hours
   c. is limited to a course of therapy no longer than 5 days
   d. often results in serious adverse reactions
8. If an antifungal agent is applied topically, the area of application is _______.
   a. washed with hydrogen peroxide before applying the antifungal drug
   b. inspected for localized skin reactions at the time of each application
   c. first covered with glycerine
   d. thoroughly scrubbed with an iodine preparation before application of the antifungal drug
9. Antifungal drugs in vaginal tablet form are inserted _______.
   a. before the patient is given a vaginal douche
   b. low in the vagina
   c. high in the vagina
10. If the patient has a ringworm infection, which of the following would be included in a patient teaching plan? _______
   a. Soak the affected area every hour while awake.
   b. Get as much exposure to sunlight as possible, as this reduces the spread of infection.
   c. Keep the infected area clean and dry.

Clinical Situation

Mrs. Joseph has an infection in her left heel which is draining a moderate amount of purulent material. She is admitted to the hospital for medical and possibly surgical treatment of the infected area.

11. Following culture and sensitivity tests, the physician prescribes clindamycin (Cleocin). Prior to the administration of the first dose of any antibiotic, the _______.
   a. patient is placed in isolation
   b. symptoms of the infection are identified and recorded
   c. patient must be seen by a physician
12. Mrs. Joseph's vital signs should be monitored _______.
   a. daily
   b. every 12 hours
   c. every 4 hours
   d. hourly
13. Mrs. Joseph should be observed for adverse drug reactions _______.
   a. at frequent intervals, especially during the first 48 hours of therapy
   b. every 12 hours during the first week of therapy
14. Therapy has proved ineffective and the antibiotic is changed to oral tetracycline. The tetracyclines, with the exception of doxycycline and minocycline, _______.
   a. may be given with food
   b. are not given with food or dairy products
   c. are given immediately after meals
   d. are given with antacids

15. The physician changes the oral tetracylcine to IM administration. The injection sites are _______.
   a. inspected weekly for signs of inflammation
   b. not rotated, since it is necessary to deposit a large amount of the drug in the extremities
   c. limited to the arms, since she has an infection in her heel
   d. rotated
16. Mrs. Joseph is experiencing a sore mouth and throat and diarrhea. The symptoms may indicate _______.
   a. an allergy to the tetracyclines
   b. the presence of a systemic infection
   c. a superinfection
   d. nephrotoxicity
17. Because of these symptoms, the nurse should _______.
   a. withhold the next dose and notify the physician
   b. continue to observe Mrs. Joseph at more frequent intervals
18. In order to evaluate Mrs. Joseph's response to therapy, the nurse should _______.
   a. monitor her vital signs daily
   b. ask Mrs. Joseph if she thinks the infection is being controlled by the antibiotic
   c. record the present symptoms and compare them with the original symptoms on a daily basis
   d. note if Mrs. Joseph's appetite has improved

III. FILL-IN AND ESSAY QUESTIONS

Read each of the following questions carefully and place your answer in the space provided.

1. Give any three points that may be included in a teaching plan for the patient taking an antibiotic following discharge from the hospital.

   1. ______________________________

      ____

   2. ______________________________

      ____

   3. ______________________________

      ____

2. To decrease the chance of noncompliance to the prescribed treatment regimen, briefly describe what can be told to the patient who has been prescribed an antibiotic for an infection.

   ____

   ____

   ____

   ____

   ____

   ____

24

Antitubercular and Leprostatic Agents

The following questions are concerned with the contents of Chapter 24, **Antitubercular and Leprostatic Agents**.

I. TRUE OR FALSE

Read each statement carefully and place your answer in the space provided.

1. __F__ Antitubercular drugs, when given in sufficient doses, cure tuberculosis.
2. __T__ Hearing testing may be performed if an antitubercular drug is known to be ototoxic.
3. __T__ Many laboratory and diagnostic tests may be necessary before starting drug therapy for tuberculosis.
4. __T__ Antitubercular drugs that cause gastric irritation can be given with food.
5. __F__ When antitubercular drugs are given parenterally, it is not necessary to rotate injection sites.
6. __T__ Although rare in the colder climates, leprosy may be seen in tropical and subtropical zones.

II. MULTIPLE CHOICE QUESTIONS

Circle the letter of the most appropriate answer.

1. Antitubercular drugs are _______.
   a. bacteriostatic b. bactericidal
2. Isoniazid may be used in the treatment of tuberculosis as well as preventive therapy in _______.
   1. household contacts of those recently diagnosed as having tuberculosis
   2. those at risk of developing tuberculosis
   3. workers in general hospitals
   4. those under age 35 with a positive skin test

   a. all but 1 b. all but 2 c. all but 3 d. all but 4
3. Treatment of tuberculosis usually involves _______.
   a. the use of a single drug
   b. keeping the patient hospitalized until the chest radiograph is clear
   c. surgical removal of all tubercular lesions
   d. the use of two or more drugs at the same time
4. In order to slow bacterial resistance to an antitubercular drug, the physician may initially prescribe _______.
   a. two or more drugs
   b. an antibiotic given with the drug
   c. the drug given every second or third day
   d. the drug given once a week

5. The most common adverse reaction associated with the administration of aminosalicylic acid (PAS) is _______.
   a. usually serious and even fatal
   b. related to the genitourinary tract
   c. related to the GI tract
   d. often due to the location of the tubercular lesion(s)

6. Antitubercular drugs are _______.
   a. administered at weekly intervals
   b. given for a long period of time
   c. rarely necessary unless the patient exhibits many symptoms of the infection
   d. only administered when the sputum is positive for the tuberculosis bacillus

7. When teaching the patient who is taking an antitubercular drug on an out-patient basis, the nurse should tell the patient _______.
   a. to double the next dose if a dose is missed
   b. to take aspirin if a fever is present
   c. not to take the drug if symptoms improve
   d. not to increase or decrease the dose unless directed to do so by the physician

8. Leprostatic drugs _______.
   a. can only be given by the parenteral route
   b. are highly toxic and can only be given for a short period of time
   c. are given orally

25

Drugs Used in the Treatment of Parasitic Infections

The following questions are concerned with the contents of Chapter 25, **Drugs Used in the Treatment of Parasitic Infections**.

I. TRUE OR FALSE

Read each statement carefully and place your answer in the space provided.

1. _______ Invasion of the body by the amoeba is called amebiasis.
2. _______ Malaria is transmitted by the *Anopheles* mosquito.
3. _______ Not all antimalarial drugs are effective in preventing or treating all of the plasmodium causing malaria.
4. _______ Most antimalarial drugs are given or taken with food or meals.
5. _______ Most helminths normally live in the stomach of the infected individual.

II. MULTIPLE CHOICE QUESTIONS

Circle the letter of the most appropriate answer.

1. The plasmodium causing malaria reproduces in _______.
   a. humans
   b. animals
   c. the mosquito
2. The symptoms of malaria appear when which one of the following events occurs in the individual bit by a mosquito carrying malaria? _______
   a. Gametocytes mate in the stomach.
   b. Plasmodium sexually reproduce.
   c. Sporozoites enter the salivary glands.
   d. Merozoites enter the red blood cells.
3. Antimalarial drugs interfere with or are active against the _______.
   a. life cycle of the plasmodium
   b. gametocycte stage of plasmodium production
   c. life cycle of the mosquito

4. When an antimalarial drug is ordered for the suppression of malaria, the drug is being used to _______.
   a. treat an active case of malaria
   b. prevent the chills and fever from becoming worse once these symptoms have occurred
   c. prevent malaria
   d. provide an immunity to malaria
5. Before an anthelmintic drug can be prescribed, the helminth must first be identified by _______.
   a. blood smears
   b. microscopic examination of the stool
   c. growing the helminth in a culture medium
6. The diagnosis of a pinworm infection is made by _______.
   a. examining the anal area and taking a specimen
   b. stool cultures
   c. blood smears
7. When a patient has a helminth infection, gloves should be worn by all personnel when _______.
   a. administering medications, taking an oral temperature
   b. changing bed linens, obtaining stool specimens
   c. bringing in the food tray, taking the blood pressure
8. Amebiasis is less common in _______.
   a. healthy individuals
   b. tropical countries
   c. areas where amebicides are available
   d. countries where sanitary facilities prevent the spread of the microorganism
9. The two types of amebiasis are _______.
   a. hepatic and splenic
   b. intestinal and pulmonary
   c. intestinal and extraintestinal
10. When a patient has amebiasis, local health departments usually require _______.
    a. hospitalization of the patient
    b. follow-up chest radiographs after treatment with an amebicide
    c. one negative stool sample following a course of treatment
    d. investigation into the source of the infection
11. Stool specimens for laboratory examination for the amoeba causing amebiasis are _______.
    a. kept refrigerated until examined
    b. taken to the laboratory immediately since the amoeba dies when the specimen cools
    c. packed in ice to preserve them before being taken to the laboratory
    d. placed in containers with a preservative
12. Isolation of the patient with amebiasis is usually _______.
    a. necessary b. not necessary
13. When the patient has amebiasis, stool precautions are usually _______.
    a. necessary b. not necessary

III. FILL-IN AND ESSAY QUESTIONS

Read each of the following questions carefully and place your answer in the space provided.

1. List or describe any five points or topics that may covered in a teaching plan for the patient with a helminth infection.

   1. ____

   ____

   2. ____

   ____

   3. ____

   ____

   4. ____

   ____

   5. ____

   ____

26

Miscellaneous Anti-Infective Drugs

The following questions are concerned with the contents of Chapter 26, **Miscellaneous Anti-Infective Drugs**.

I. TRUE OR FALSE

Read each statement carefully and place your answer in the space provided.

1. ______ There are very few drugs available for the treatment of some types of viral infections.
2. ______ Some antiviral agents appear to inhibit the manufacture of glucose by a virus.
3. ______ Acyclovir (Zovirax) is effective against the common cold.
4. ______ Amantadine (Symmetrel) is used for the prevention or treatment of influenza A virus respiratory tract illness in high-risk patients.
5. ______ Urinary anti-infectives not belonging to the antibiotic or sulfonamide group of drugs exert their antibacterial effects in the urine.
6. ______ Furazolidone (Furoxone) is used in the treatment of diarrhea resulting from certain strains of bacteria or protozoa.
7. ______ An antiseptic stops, slows, or prevents the growth of microorganisms.
8. ______ Iodine solutions do not permanently stain clothing and other objects.
9. ______ Merbromin and thimerosal contain mercury.
10. ______ A germicide is an agent that kills bacteria.

II. MULTIPLE CHOICE QUESTIONS

Circle the letter of the most appropriate answer.

1. In addition to its use as an antiviral agent, amantadine is also used in the treatment of ______.
   a. Parkinson's disease
   b. pneumonia in the newborn
   c. staphylococcal pneumonia
   d. hepatitis
2. Zidovudine (AZT) is used in the treatment of ______.
   a. viral encephalitis
   b. herpes zoster
   c. AIDS and ARC
   d. infectious mononucleosis
3. Acute or chronic pulmonary reactions may be seen with the administration of nitrofurantoin (Furadantin) and are manifested by ______.
   a. malaise, hypothermia, muscle pain or tenderness
   b. dyspnea, chest pain, cough
   c. tachycardia, chest pain, decreased respiratory rate

4. Which one of the following tasks should be performed by the nurse when the patient is receiving a urinary anti-infective? _______
   a. Limit the patient's fluid intake.
   b. Test the urine for glucose and ketones every 2 hours.
   c. Obtain a urine sample for culture and sensitivity daily.
   d. Monitor the vital signs every 4 hours.
5. Systemic urinary anti-infective drugs _______.
   a. are given on an empty stomach to enhance absorption
   b. should be given with food or meals to prevent gastrointestinal upset
6. Nitrofurantoin and methenamine work best in _______ urine.
   a. acid   b. alkaline
7. Pentamidine isothionate (Pentam 300) is used in the treatment or prevention of __d__.
   a. influenza A and B
   b. herpes zoster
   c. herpes simplex viral encephalitis
   d. *Pneumocystis carinii* pneumonia
8. Furazolidone (Furoxone) _______ affects the normal bacterial flora of the intestine.
   a. does   b. does not
9. The action of topical germicides and antiseptics may depend on the _______.
   a. type of dressing applied after application
   b. strength of the drug
   c. patient
10. Povidone-iodine is often preferred over iodine because it is _______.
    a. stronger and more effective
    b. colorless
    c. less irritating to the skin
11. Topical antiseptics and germicides are primarily used to _______.
    a. reduce the number of bacteria on skin surfaces
    b. sterilize the skin
12. Ophthalmic ointments are applied to the _______.
    a. upper conjunctival sac
    b. eyelids or lower conjunctival sac
13. Ophthalmic solutions are dropped into the _______.
    a. inner corner (canthus) of the eye
    b. lower conjunctival sac

III. FILL-IN AND ESSAY QUESTIONS

Read each of the following questions carefully and place your answer in the space provided.

1. List or describe any three areas or points that may be included in a teaching plan for the patient taking a systemic anti-infective for a urinary tract infection.
   1. Take the drug c̄ food or meals (nitrofurantoin
   2. Take drugs at the intervals prescribe by the physician
   3. Notify physician immediately if symptoms does not improve within 3 - 4 days
2. Briefly explain why anxiety might be stated as a nursing diagnosis when the patient is receiving pentamidine isothionate?

   anxiety may be R/T diagnosis & prognosis because the drug is given to those with aids

3. List any four uses of ophthalmic or otic preparations.
   1. eye infection, eye pain or inflammation
   2. treatment of glaucoma, preparation of eye surgery
   3. ear infection, ear pain, inflammation of the
   4. auditory cannal

4. List or describe any four areas or points that are included in a teaching plan for the patient prescribed an ophthalmic preparation.

1. Wash hands thoroughly before cleansing the eyelids instilling eye drops, or applying an eye ointment
2. Instill the prescribed number of drops or amount of ointment in the eye.
3. Complete a full course of treatment with the prescribed drug to achieve satisfactory results
4. Do not rub the eyes & keep hands away from the eye

IV. Discussion*

1. AIDS (acquired immunodeficiency syndrome) and ARC (AIDS related complex) are two serious health problems. Health personnel must exert special care in order to prevent the spread of AIDS as well as protect themselves from this fatal infection. Suggestions for areas or topics that may be discussed include:
   - Should all individuals admitted to the hospital be screened for AIDS antibodies? If so, why is this justified?
   - What are some of the dangers associated with the screening of all patients admitted to the hospital?
   - Why might screening of all hospitalized patients be ineffective in identifying those with AIDS?
   - What are some of the methods that may be used by the general public and by health care workers to prevent the spread of AIDS?
   - Can public education reduce the incidence of AIDS?
   - Should school children at the elementary level be taught facts about AIDS?
   - Consider the fact that in past years many hospitals required a VDRL or Wasserman—which are screening tests for syphilis—on all new admissions. Why is this different than screening all new admissions for AIDS?

*Note: Additional reading may be necessary to discuss these issues.

27

Pituitary and Adrenal Cortical Hormones

The following questions are concerned with the contents of Chapter 27, **Pituitary and Adrenal Cortical Hormones**.

I. TRUE OR FALSE

Read each statement carefully and place your answer in the space provided.

1. _______ The pituitary gland is protected by the maxillary bone.
2. _______ Menotropins is a drug used to induce ovulation and pregnancy in the anovulatory female.
3. _______ Height and weight measurements are used to evaluate the results of therapy with growth hormone.
4. _______ Glucocorticoids are not essential to life.
5. _______ The mineralocorticoids influence fat and protein metabolism.
6. _______ One function of the glucocorticoids is regulation of the immune response system.
7. _______ *Exogenous* means "produced by the body."
8. _______ Aldosterone is a mineralocorticoid.
9. _______ A deficiency of the mineralocorticoids results in a loss of potassium and retention of sodium.
10. _______ Fludrocortisone (Florinef) has both glucocorticoid and mineralocorticoid activity.
11. _______ Adrenocorticotropic hormone may be used for the diagnostic testing of adrenal cortical function.

II. MULTIPLE CHOICE QUESTIONS

Circle the letter of the most appropriate answer.

1. Follicle-stimulating hormone and luteinizing hormone are called _______.
   a. menotropins
   b. posterior pituitary hormones
   c. chorionic hormones
   d. gonadotropins
2. The growth hormone secreted by the anterior pituitary is also called _______.
   a. luteotrophic hormone
   b. somatotrophic hormone
   c. prolactin
   d. menotrophic hormone

3. Growth hormone, which is given to those who have failed to grow, can only be administered _______.
   a. prior to closure of the bone epiphyses
   b. after closure of the bone epiphyses
4. Adrenocorticotropic hormone (ACTH) _______.
   a. stimulates the adrenal medulla to secrete epinephrine
   b. controls the activity of the pituitary gland
   c. stimulates the adrenal cortex to produce and secrete adrenal cortical hormones
   d. is produced by the posterior pituitary
5. Vasopressin _______.
   a. promotes the reabsorption of water by the kidneys
   b. suppresses the posterior pituitary
   c. controls electrolyte balance by direct action on the kidneys
   d. encourages the loss of water by the kidneys
6. Vasopressin is used in the treatment of _______.
   a. diabetes mellitus
   b. diabetes insipidus
   c. electrolyte imbalances
   d. dehydration
7. Following administration of vasopressin, the patient is observed every 10 to 15 minutes for signs of overdose which may include _______.
   a. excessive urinary output
   b. nausea, diarrhea, excessive perspiration
   c. dry skin, flushing, hypothermia
   d. blanching of the skin, nausea, abdominal cramps
8. Which of the following nursing measures are instituted when vasopressin is administered for diabetes insipidus? _______
   a. accurate intake and output, observation for signs of a fluid volume deficit or fluid overload
   b. weekly weights, blood pressure every 8 hours
   c. auscultation of the abdomen, limiting the patient's fluid intake
   d. forcing fluids, encouraging a high protein diet
9. The two most prominent glucocorticoids produced by the adrenal gland are _______.
   a. cortisol and corticotropin
   b. adrenocorticotropin and sex hormones
   c. cortisone and corticol
   d. cortisone and hydrocortisone
10. The mineralocoticoids play an important role in _______.
   a. promoting the release of ACTH from the pituitary
   b. glucose metabolism
   c. conserving sodium and increasing the excretion of potassium
   d. promoting the secretion of aldosterone

Clinical Situation

Mrs. Bateman has severe rheumatoid arthritis, which has not responded well to therapy with anti-inflammatory agents. Her physician now prescribes a glucocorticoid, in an attempt to prevent further joint destruction as well as relieve the symptoms of the disorder.

11. Administration of a glucocorticoid to Mrs. Bateman over a period of as little as 5 to 10 days will result in _______.
   a. drug tolerance
   b. increasing the amount of endogenous glucocorticoids secreted by the adrenal gland
   c. shutting off the pituitary release of ACTH
   d. drug sensitivity
12. When the adrenals fail to manufacture and release glucocorticoids, the _______.
   a. pituitary will enlarge
   b. patient has acute adrenal insufficiency
   c. patient has an excess of endogenous adrenal hormones
   d. adrenals will enlarge
13. The response of the pituitary to high or low levels of glucocorticoids and the resulting release or nonrelease of ACTH is an example of _______.
   a. acute adrenal insufficiency
   b. adrenal shutdown
   c. the feedback mechanism
   d. the shutdown mechanism
14. Mrs. Bateman will need to be observed for the adverse effects of glucocorticoid administration, which include _______.
   1. sodium and fluid retention
   2. potassium retention
   3. hyperglycemia
   4. osteoporosis
   5. hypertension

   a. 1, 2, 3 b. 2, 3, 4 c. 2, 4, 5 d. 1, 4, 5
15. Mrs. Bateman must be observed for signs of electrolyte imbalance. Which of the following imbalances might occur in this patient? _______
   a. hypernatremia, hypokalemia
   b. hypercalcemia, hyperkalemia
   c. respiratory acidosis, hyponatremia

16. Nursing personnel and visitors with any type of infection should avoid contact with Mrs. Bateman because _______.
    a. she may be a carrier for bacteria normally found in a hospital
    b. of her possible decreased resistance to infection
    c. glucocorticoid administration increases the white blood cell count
    d. she has an infectious form of arthritis
17. Mrs. Bateman also has diabetes mellitus which is controlled with insulin. While on glucocorticoid therapy, she may require _______.
    a. a diet high in carbohydrates and low in proteins
    b. testing of her urine for glucose every 2 hours
    c. frequent adjustment in her insulin dosage
    d. approximately one half her usual daily dose of insulin
18. If Mrs. Bateman was not a diabetic, her urine would still be checked for glucose once a week because the glucocorticoids may _______.
    a. cause false-positive urine tests for glucose
    b. increase the excretion of ketones
    c. cause diabetes
    d. aggravate latent diabetes
19. After 3 weeks the physician has decided to discontinue glucocorticoid therapy. Discontinuation of therapy is accomplished by _______.
    a. tapering the dose over a period of days
    b. abruptly discontinuing the drug
20. The answer to question 19 is based on the fact that _______.
    a. abrupt discontinuation of these drugs can result in acute adrenal insufficiency
    b. glucocorticoids must be discontinued abruptly to allow the pituitary to begin secreting ACTH

III. FILL-IN AND ESSAY QUESTIONS

Read each of the following questions carefully and place your answer in the space provided.

1. The two hormones produced by the posterior pituitary gland are ____________________ and ____________________.
2. Briefly explain the alternate-day therapy regimen for the administration of a glucocorticoid. Include in the explanation the time(s) of day the drug is given as well as the rationale for giving the drug at the selected time(s).

    ____

    ____

    ____

    ____

    ____

3. Describe or list any five points that can be included in a teaching plan for the patient prescribed long-term or high-dose glucocorticoid therapy.

    1. ____

    ____

    2. ____

    ____

    3. ____

    ____

    4. ____

    ____

    5. ____

    ____

28

Male and Female Hormones

The following questions are concerned with the contents of Chapter 28, **Male and Female Hormones**.

I. TRUE OR FALSE

Read each statement carefully and place your answer in the space provided.

1. _______ The production of male and female hormones is under the influence of the anterior pituitary gland.
2. _______ Small amounts of male and female hormones are produced by the adrenal cortex.
3. _______ Anabolic steroids may be used to help the patient lose weight.
4. _______ Anabolic steroids are closely related to the estrogens.
5. _______ Only estrogens are used as oral contraceptives.

II. MULTIPLE CHOICE QUESTIONS

Circle the letter of the most appropriate answer.

1. Tissue-building processes, which are promoted by the androgens, are also called _______.
   a. anabolism b. catabolism
2. Tissue-depleting processes, which are reversed by the androgens, are also called _______.
   a. anabolism b. catabolism
3. Androgen therapy may be used in females with inoperable metastatic breast cancer who _______.
   a. have not had an oophorectomy
   b. do not wish to have radiation treatments
   c. are 1 to 5 years past menopause
   d. have not had chemotherapy
4. Hormone-dependent tumors in the female are malignancies that _______.
   a. require estrogen therapy to halt their growth and spread
   b. grow and spread under the influence of estrogen
   c. require progesterone therapy to counteract the effect of estrogen on the tumor
   d. grow and spread under the influence of androgens
5. Anabolic steroids may be used in the _______.
   a. management of osteoporosis occurring past menopause
   b. treatment of iron-deficiency anemia
   c. management of profound anabolism
   d. treatment of growth failure

6. The most common adverse reactions to androgens in the female are _______.
   a. menopausal symptoms, nausea
   b. weight loss, hypotension
   c. hair loss, hyponatremia
   d. menstrual irregularities, virilization
7. The most potent estrogen is _______.
   a. estrane
   b. estradiol
   c. estriol
   d. progesterone
8. Estrogens are secreted by the _______.
   a. anterior pituitary
   b. endometrium
   c. ovarian follicle
   d. corpus luteum
9. Progesterone is secreted by the _______.
   a. anterior pituitary
   b. corpus luteum
   c. endometrium
   d. fallopian tubes
10. Which of the following are uses of the estrogens? _______
    1. management of inoperable prostatic carcinoma
    2. relief of postpartum breast engorgement
    3. management of the symptoms of menopause
    4. as oral contraceptives

    a. 1, 3 b. 2, 3 c. 1, 4 d. all of these
11. Progestins are primarily used in the treatment of _______.
    a. amenorrhea, functional uterine bleeding
    b. ovarian or breast carcinoma
    c. menopause, breast carcinoma
    d. dysmenorrhea, premenstrual syndrome
12. When a patient is using an oral contraceptive, cigarette smoking increases the risk of _______.
    a. ovarian carcinoma
    b. extreme weight loss
    c. cardiovascular side effects such as thromboembolism
    d. marked hypotension
13. An oral contraceptive is best taken _______.
    a. early in the morning before breakfast
    b. with the evening meal or at bedtime
    c. during or after the noon meal
14. The effectiveness of an oral contraceptive depends on _______.
    a. the brand of drug prescribed
    b. taking the drug on an empty stomach
    c. following the prescribed dosage schedule

III. FILL-IN AND ESSAY QUESTIONS

Read each of the following questions carefully and place your answer in the space provided.

1. Male hormones are called ____________________.
2. The female hormones are ____________________ and ____________________.
3. List or describe any three signs of virilization in the female that may be seen during androgen therapy.
   1. ____________________
   2. ____________________
   3. ____________________
4. List any three points that can be included in a teaching plan for the patient taking an estrogen or progestin.
   1. ____________________
   2. ____________________
   3. ____________________
5. List or describe any three points that can be included in a teaching plan for the patient taking an oral contraceptive.
   1. ____________________

2. ____

____

3. ____

____

6. The use of anabolic steroids by healthy individuals to increase muscle mass poses serious risks. List any three serious adverse reactions that may be seen with prolonged high-dose use of the anabolic steroids for this purpose.

1. ____
2. ____
3. ____

29

Thyroid and Antithyroid Drugs

The following questions are concerned with the contents of Chapter 29, **Thyroid and Antithyroid Drugs**.

I. TRUE OR FALSE

Read each statement carefully and place your answer in the space provided.

1. _______ The thyroid gland is located behind the trachea.
2. _______ The activity of the thyroid gland is regulated by the posterior pituitary gland.
3. _______ Thyroid hormones influence every organ and tissue of the body.
4. _______ Hypothyroidism is due to an increase in the amount of thyroid hormones manufactured by the thyroid gland.
5. _______ The dose of thyroid hormones must be carefully adjusted according to the patient's hormone requirements.

II. MULTIPLE CHOICE QUESTIONS

Circle the letter of the most appropriate answer.

1. The activity of the thyroid gland is regulated by the _______.
   a. thyroid stimulating hormone produced by the anterior pituitary
   b. thyroid depressing hormone produced by the posterior pituitary
   c. thyroid gland itself
2. The release or nonrelease of hormones by the thyroid gland is dependent on the _______.
   a. level of iodine in the blood
   b. activity of the posterior pituitary
   c. activity of the adrenal cortex
   d. level of circulating thyroid hormones
3. Thyroid hormones are principally concerned with _______.
   a. decreasing the metabolic rate
   b. control of catabolism
   c. increasing the metabolic rate of tissues
   d. the utilization of starches in the diet
4. Antithyroid drugs _______.
   a. inhibit the release of thyroid hormones
   b. render ineffective the thyroid hormones circulating in the bloodstream
   c. inhibit the manufacture of thyroid hormones
   d. prevent iodine from entering the thyroid gland
5. Antithyroid drugs may be used in the treatment of _______.
   a. hypothyroidism
   b. hyperthyroidism

6. Thyrotoxicosis is a state of severe _______.
   a. iodine deficiency
   b. hypothyroidism
   c. thyroid gland failure
   d. hyperthyroidism
7. The most serious adverse reaction associated with methimazole (Tapazole) and propylthiouracil is _______.
   a. agranulocytosis
   b. iron-deficiency anemia
   c. hypotension
   d. an increase in the red blood cell count
8. The symptoms of iodism, which may occur with the use of iodine preparations, include _______.
   1. swelling and soreness of the parotid glands
   2. burning of the mouth and throat
   3. sore teeth and gums
   4. symptoms of a head cold

   a. 1, 2, 3 b. 1 only c. 2, 3, 4 d. all of these
9. Iodine solutions have a strong salty taste which can be partially disguised by adding the drug to _______.
   a. fruit juice b. water c. cereal

Clinical Situation

Mrs. Laver has been diagnosed as being hypothyroid and her physician has prescribed a thyroid hormone.

10. The use of a thyroid hormone for Mrs. Laver is an attempt to _______.
    a. change the iodine uptake of the thyroid gland
    b. create a euthyroid state
    c. increase the manufacture of endogenous thyroid hormones
11. During initial therapy the most common adverse reaction Mrs. Laver may experience is _______.
    a. skin rash
    b. the Stevens-Johnson syndrome
    c. peripheral edema
    d. signs of hyperthyroidism
12. Thyroid hormones are generally taken _______.
    a. with an antithyroid preparation
    b. once a day before retiring
    c. with the noon meal
    d. once a day, preferably before breakfast
13. Mrs. Laver should be told that the full effects of thyroid therapy may not be evident for _______.
    a. 24 to 48 hours
    b. 1 to 3 days
    c. several weeks or more
    d. 9 to 12 months
14. Which of the following may indicate that Mrs. Laver is responding well to therapy? _______
    a. weight gain, improvement in appetite, decrease in blood pressure
    b. weight loss, mild diuresis, sense of well-being
    c. decrease in anxiety, increase in blood pressure, regular menses
    d. decrease in pulse rate, decrease in metabolism, absence of tremors

III. FILL-IN AND ESSAY QUESTIONS

Read each of the following questions carefully and place your answer in the space provided.

1. List or describe five symptoms of hypothyroidism and hyperthyroidism.

Hypothyroidism

1. ______________________________
2. ______________________________
3. ______________________________
4. ______________________________
5. ______________________________

Hyperthyroidism

1. ______________________________
2. ______________________________
3. ______________________________
4. ______________________________
5. ______________________________

2. List or describe any three points to include in a teaching plan for Mrs. Laver, who is prescribed a thyroid drug for hypothyroidism.

1. ____

____

2. ____

____

3. ____

____

30

Drugs Acting on the Uterus

The following questions are concerned with the contents of Chapter 30, **Drugs Acting on the Uterus**.

I. TRUE OR FALSE

Read each statement carefully and place your answer in the space provided.

1. _______ Oxytocin is an endogenous hormone produced by the posterior pituitary gland.
2. _______ Ergonovine (Ergotrate) may be given to encourage postpartum relaxation of the uterus.
3. _______ The patient may complain of abdominal cramping with the use of ergonovine or methylergonovine (Methergine).
4. _______ Patients receiving IV oxytocin (Pitocin) rarely require constant supervision and observation.
5. _______ Sodium chloride 20% is an abortifacient.

II. MULTIPLE CHOICE QUESTIONS

Circle the letter of the most appropriate answer.

1. Ergonovine and methylergonovine are given _______.
   a. to induce an abortion
   b. before contractions are 2 to 3 minutes apart
   c. after the delivery of the placenta
   d. to induce labor
2. Intravenous oxytocin may be used to _______.
   a. start or improve labor contractions
   b. encourage the release of endogenous oxytocin
   c. prevent uterine bleeding during pregnancy
   d. suppress the milk ejection reflex
3. Adverse reactions associated with the use of ergonovine and methylergonovine include _______.
   1. an elevation of the blood pressure
   2. temporary chest pain
   3. headache
   4. uterine relaxation

   a. all but 1 b. all but 2 c. all but 3 d. all but 4
4. Adverse reactions associated with the use of oxytocin include _______.
   1. fetal bradycardia
   2. uterine relaxation
   3. uterine rupture
   4. maternal jaundice
   5. cardiac dysrhythmias

   a. 1, 4, 5 b. 1, 3, 5 c. 2, 4, 5 d. all of these

5. Intravenous oxytocin is best administered _______.
   a. by means of an IV infusion pump
   b. as an intermittent IV push
   c. by IV push
   d. undiluted
6. When IV oxytocin is given, which of the following requires contacting the physician immediately? _______
   1. uterine contractions lasting 5 to 10 seconds
   2. any significant change in the fetal heart rate
   3. any marked change in the rhythm of uterine contractions
   4. a urinary output of 50 mL per hour
   5. uterine contractions 5 minutes apart

   a. 1, 2 b. 2, 3 c. 3, 4 d. 4, 5
7. Intramuscular oxytocin may be given during the third stage of labor to _______.
   a. slow the delivery of the placenta
   b. encourage uterine atony
   c. stimulate the milk-ejection reflex
   d. produce uterine contractions and control postpartum bleeding and hemorrhage
8. Ritodrine (Yutopar), a uterine relaxant, is used in the management of _______.
   a. postpartum bleeding
   b. postabortion bleeding
   c. preterm labor
   d. difficult placental deliveries
9. Following insertion of an IV line for administration of ritodrine, the patient is usually placed in a _______ position.
   a. left lateral b. prone c. supine
10. The abortifacients carboprost (Prostin/15 M) and dinoprostone (Prostin E2) _______.
    a. increase the production of oxytocin by the pituitary
    b. stimulate the uterus to contract
    c. decrease uterine contractions and increase uterine muscle tone
    d. act on the placenta
11. Carboprost and dinoprostone are normally used to abort the fetus after approximately the _______ week of pregnancy.
    a. third to fifth
    b. twelfth to thirteenth
    c. twenty-eighth to thirtieth
12. A transabdominal tap is necessary for the administration of _______.
    a. carboprost
    b. dinoprostone
    c. sodium chloride
13. Following administration of an abortifacient, the patient is observed for the onset of uterine contractions every _______.
    a. 5 minutes
    b. 30 minutes to 1 hour
    c. 8 hours
    d. day

III. FILL-IN AND ESSAY QUESTIONS

Read each of the following questions carefully and place your answer in the space provided.

1. List any three nursing assessments made immediately prior to starting an IV infusion of oxytocin.
   1. ______________________________
   2. ______________________________
   3. ______________________________
2. List any four observations and assessments made following administration of an abortifacient.
   1. ______________________________
   2. ______________________________
   3. ______________________________
   4. ______________________________

IV. Discussion

1. Discuss the emotional needs that may be encountered when a patient is having an abortion and how the nurse may try to deal with the patient's needs before, during, and after the abortion procedure.

31

Antineoplastic Drugs

The following questions are concerned with the contents of Chapter 31, **Antineoplastic Drugs**.

I. TRUE OR FALSE

Read each statement carefully and place your answer in the space provided.

1. _______ Antineoplastic drugs are used in the treatment of malignant diseases.
2. _______ The antineoplastic antibiotics also have anti-infective activity.
3. _______ Antineoplastic drugs produce a wide variety of adverse reactions.
4. _______ The dose of some antineoplastic agents may be based on the patient's weight.
5. _______ The patient's response to an antineoplastic drug is predictable.
6. _______ Patients receiving chemotherapy can be at different stages of the malignant disease.
7. _______ Knowing what adverse reactions will occur allows the nurse to prepare for any events that may happen.
8. _______ Patients should be told about the adverse reactions that may occur during therapy with an antineoplastic drug.
9. _______ An antiemetic may be given prior to the administration of an antineoplastic drug known to cause severe vomiting.
10. _______ Alopecia is the excessive growth of hair on the face.

II. MULTIPLE CHOICE QUESTIONS

Circle the letter of the most appropriate answer.

Clinical Situation

Mrs. Langly, age 41, is admitted to the oncology unit of the hospital for chemotherapy.

1. Antineoplastic drugs _______.
   a. may slow the rate of tumor growth and delay metastasis
   b. cure most malignant diseases when given in large doses
   c. change tumor cells into nonmalignant cells
2. Generally, antineoplastic drugs affect _______.
   a. only malignant cells
   b. cells that rapidly proliferate
   c. only superficial cancer cells
   d. cells that slowly proliferate
3. Antineoplastic drugs _______.
   a. are given as single drugs only
   b. may be given in combination with other antineoplastic drugs
   c. work best when two drugs are given a week apart

4. Some of the adverse reactions that may be seen when Mrs. Langly receives chemotherapy _______.
   a. can be treated with other antineoplastic drugs
   b. may be less serious because of her age group
   c. may be dose-dependent
   d. can be lessened by increasing the initial dosage
5. While Mrs. Langly is receiving chemotherapy, the nurse should remember that _______.
   a. the occurrence of serious adverse reactions is rare
   b. these drugs are not toxic when given in recommended doses
   c. the development of adverse reactions almost always depends on the type of malignancy being treated
   d. these drugs are potentially toxic
6. Mrs. Langly is to be given cisplatin (Platinol). Prior to administration of this drug, Mrs. Langly will be _______.
   a. placed in isolation
   b. given enemas until clear
   c. hydrated with 1 to 2 liters of IV fluid
   d. placed in reverse isolation
7. When preparing the parenteral forms of antineoplastic drugs, the nurse must _______.
   a. wear plastic disposable gloves
   b. avoid touching the outside of the bottle once the diluent is added
   c. prepare the drug 24 hours before use
8. Which of the following will influence the nursing management of Mrs. Langly? _______
   1. her general physical condition
   2. adverse reactions that may occur
   3. her response to the drug
   4. guidelines established by the hospital
   5. results of periodic laboratory tests

   a. all of these b. 1, 2, 5 c. 2, 3, 4 d. 3, 4, 5
9. The other patient in the room with Mrs. Langly is Mrs. Stevens, who is receiving melphalan (Alkeran). One adverse reaction associated with the administration of this drug is hyperuricemia. When this reaction is known to occur, the patient will be _______.
   a. placed in reverse isolation
   b. watched for signs of pulmonary edema
   c. assessed for changes in the heart rate
   d. encouraged to drink at least 2000 mL of water per day
10. Mrs. Langly is allowed to ambulate and meets another patient, Miss Agronsky, in the hallway. Mrs. Langly notes that the patient has lost most of her hair. Nurses should consider alopecia to be a _______.
    a. minor problem that is no cause for concern, as the hair will grow back
    b. personal problem that is best not to mention
    c. serious problem, since the hair will not grow back
    d. personal problem that may cause great emotional concern on the part of the patient
11. If Mrs. Langly has a significant drop in her platelet count, nursing measures would include _______.
    a. observing her daily for signs of increased urinary output
    b. watching for signs of electrolyte imbalance
    c. the prevention of bleeding and bruising episodes
    d. placing her in isolation
12. Mrs. Langly has frequent blood counts, which are necessary to _______.
    a. monitor her response to a diet high in iron
    b. determine the bone marrow depressing effect of the antineoplastic drug
    c. determine if she has an infection

III. FILL-IN AND ESSAY QUESTIONS

Read each of the following questions carefully and place your answer in the space provided.

1. List or describe any four initial nursing assessments that should be made prior to starting chemotherapy.

   1. ______________________________
   2. ______________________________
   3. ______________________________
   4. ______________________________

2. List or decribe any five general points or areas that can be included in a teaching plan for the patient taking an oral antineoplastic drug on an outpatient basis.

   1. ______________________________

   ____

2. ______________________________

3. ______________________________

4. ______________________________

5. ______________________________

IV. DISCUSSION

1. Patients with a malignant disease need special consideration, understanding, and emotional support. On occasion, these needs are unrecognized by members of the medical profession. If you were recently diagnosed as having cancer, what would be some of the feelings you would experience at this time? What would you want the nurse to do for you at this time? What would be your thoughts about your future? What would you want to know or not know? As you think about or discuss these questions, remember that any patient may have these same emotional responses and may need the same things you would expect from the nurse or other members of the medical profession.

32

Anticonvulsant Drugs

The following questions are concerned with the contents of Chapter 32, **Anticonvulsant Drugs**.

I. TRUE OR FALSE

Read each statement carefully and place your answer in the space provided.

1. _______ Epilepsy is a term applied to a permanent recurrent seizure disorder.
2. _______ Epileptic seizures are characterized by a specific pattern of events.
3. _______ If one anticonvulsant does not control seizures, it is unlikely that another anticonvulsant will be of value.
4. _______ Idiopathic epilepsy has a known cause.
5. _______ Electrolyte imbalances may cause a seizure.

II. MULTIPLE CHOICE QUESTIONS

Circle the letter of the most appropriate answer.

1. Generally, the anticonvulsants _______.
   a. increase the excitability of the neurons of the brain
   b. stabilize the neurons in the spinal cord
   c. reduce the excitability of the neurons of the brain
   d. act on all nerve cells in the body
2. Which of the following may be causes of an acquired seizure disorder? _______
   1. high fever
   2. uremia
   3. brain tumors
   4. moderate hypotension

   a. 1, 2, 3 b. 2, 3, 4 c. 2 only d. 1, 3
3. Which of the following should be noted when a patient has a seizure? _______
   1. time of occurrence
   2. length of the seizure
   3. psychic or motor activity during the seizure
   4. the ability of the patient to terminate his or her seizure

   a. all but 1 b. all but 2 c. all but 3 d. all but 4
4. Abrupt withdrawal of an anticonvulsant can result in _______.
   a. having to restart the medication at a higher dose
   b. a decreased response to any anticonvulsant
   c. status epilepticus
   d. having to use a different anticonvulsant
5. Until seizures are controlled _______.
   a. some activities may need to be limited
   b. the patient must be hospitalized
   c. the patient will require at least two anticonvulsants given together
   d. the patient can do anything she or he wishes except drive a car

Clinical Situation

Mr. O'Brien, age 25, has epilepsy which was diagnosed when he was 2 years old.

6. Mr. O'Brien tells you that he has had several dosage adjustments of his anticonvulsant drug over the past 4 years. Dosage adjustments may be necessary _______.
   a. when the patient is over age 20
   b. during periods of stress
7. When taking a drug history, Mr. O'Brien tells you that he originally was given metharbital (Gemonil), a barbiturate. The most common adverse reaction seen with the barbiturate anticonvulsants is _______.
   a. sedation b. vomiting c. skin rash d. diarrhea
8. Through the years Mr. O'Brien has been prescribed various anticonvulsants. Presently he is taking phenytoin (Dilantin), one of the hydantoins. The most common adverse reaction seen with this group of drugs is related to the _______.
   a. liver and pancreas
   b. GU tract
   c. central nervous system
   d. lower GI tract
9. Mr. O'Brien was told to see his dentist frequently, as the hydantoins may cause _______.
   a. cavities
   b. staining of the teeth
   c. oral tumors
   d. gingival hyperplasia
10. When Mr. O'Brien was first diagnosed at age 2, the reason his parents probably sought medical attention was his abnormal behavior pattern or convulsive movements. At that time a thorough patient history would have been important to _______.
    a. determine if the seizures could be cured
    b. identify the type of seizure disorder
    c. determine if drug therapy would control the seizures
11. Mr. O'Brien also states that his parents told him that many diagnostic tests were done after they first saw a physician. These tests would have been done to _______.
    a. confirm the diagnosis and provide a baseline during therapy
    b. see if another seizure would occur
    c. determine which drug would work best
12. Mr. O'Brien tells you that his anticonvulsant causes nausea. At this point it will be important to determine if Mr. O'Brien _______.
    a. thinks another drug should be tried
    b. drinks extra water during the day
    c. is telling the truth
    d. takes the drug with food

III. FILL-IN AND ESSAY QUESTIONS

Read each of the following questions carefully and place your answer in the space provided.

1. Develop a teaching plan covering the following points for the newly diagnosed epileptic.
   a. Taking the medication. ______________________________

   ____

   b. Carrying identification. ______________________________

   ____

   c. Use of nonprescription drugs. ______________________________

   ____

   d. Drinking. ______________________________

   ____

   e. Local agencies that can offer information and assistance. ______________________________

   ____

33

Antiparkinsonism Drugs

The following questions are concerned with the contents of Chapter 33, **Antiparkinsonism Drugs**.

I. TRUE OR FALSE

Read each statement carefully and place your answer in the space provided.

1. _______ Another name for Parkinson's disease is paralysis agitans.
2. _______ Parkinsonism is a term that refers to the symptoms of Parkinson's disease as well as parkinsonlike symptoms due to other causes.
3. _______ A monotone speech pattern may be seen in the patient with parkinsonism.
4. _______ Patients with parkinsonism rarely have mental changes.

II. MULTIPLE CHOICE QUESTIONS

Circle the letter of the most appropriate answer.

1. Parkinson's disease is thought to be due to a deficiency of _______.
   a. dopamine in the CNS
   b. acetylcholine and acetylcholinesterase in the CNS
   c. dopamine in peripheral nerve fibers
   d. norepinephrine in the CNS
2. Which of the following are some of the signs and symptoms of Parkinson's disease that may be noted during the nursing assessment? _______
   1. excessive or abnormal hair loss
   2. masklike facial expression
   3. difficulty in chewing and swallowing
   4. shuffling gait
   5. paralysis

   a. 1, 2, 5 b. 1, 4, 5 c. 2, 3, 4 d. 3, 4, 5
3. Antiparkinsonism drugs with anticholinergic activity _______.
   a. inhibit acetylcholine
   b. increase dopamine manufacture
   c. increase norepinephrine release
   d. inhibit acetylcholinesterase
4. Carbidopa (Lodosyn) _______.
   a. is the most potent antiparkinsonism drug
   b. must be given with levodopa (Larodopa)
   c. is more toxic than levodopa (Larodopa)
5. Selegiline (Eldepryl) is usually used for those _______.
   a. with a mild form of parkinsonism
   b. taking an anticholinergic antiparkinsonism drug
   c. requiring special diets
   d. not responding to therapy with carbidopa and levodopa

6. Levodopa (Larodopa) is _______.
   a. less effective than dopamine
   b. a metabolic precursor of dopamine
   c. cannot be given with carbidopa
   d. less effective than drugs with anticholinergic activity

Clinical Situation

Mrs. Adler, age 81, has had Parkinson's disease for 14 years.

7. Mrs. Adler has been taking an anticholinergic antiparkinsonism drug. Adverse reactions frequently seen with these drugs include _______.
   a. constipation, urinary frequency, loss of peripheral vision
   b. nausea, hypotension, muscle spasms
   c. diarrhea, hypertension, bradycardia
   d. dry mouth, blurred vision, dizziness
8. The physician has decided to discontinue Mrs. Adler's present drug and start her on levodopa. The most serious and frequent adverse reactions seen with levodopa include _______.
   a. tachycardia and hypotension
   b. choreiform and dystonic movements
   c. excessive salivation and convulsions
   d. dry mouth and urinary retention
9. A less frequent but serious adverse reaction to levodopa is _______.
   a. mental changes such as depression and psychotic episodes
   b. cardiac dysrhythmias such as paroxysmal tachycardia
   c. GI upset such as constipation
   d. CNS reactions such as a decrease in tremors
10. Why is it important to watch Mrs. Adler closely for adverse reactions? _______
    a. Some patients with parkinsonism communicate poorly and will not tell the nurse that problems are occurring.
    b. The drug she is taking causes extreme sedation.
11. Mrs. Adler has had a sudden change in her behavior. This should _______.
    a. not cause concern as it is part of Parkinson's disease
    b. cause concern since it may be an adverse reaction

III. FILL-IN AND ESSAY QUESTIONS

Read each of the following questions carefully and place your answer in the space provided.

1. The patient's neurological status is evaluated prior to starting therapy with an antiparkinsonism drug. List or describe any five signs and symptoms of parkinsonism that may be seen during a neurological assessment.

   1. ____________________
   2. ____________________
   3. ____________________
   4. ____________________
   5. ____________________

2. In recent years, Mrs. Wilson's parkinsonism has resulted in injury from falls and other accidents. She has moved from her home and she will now be living with her daughter. What suggestions can be made to Mrs. Wilson's daughter to make her home more safe and least likely to result in accidents or falls?

   ____

   ____

   ____

   ____

   ____

34

Psychotherapeutic Drugs

The following questions are concerned with the contents of Chapter 34, **Psychotherapeutic Drugs**.

I. TRUE OR FALSE

Read each statement carefully and place your answer in the space provided.

1. _______ A drug that affects the mind is called a psychotropic drug.
2. _______ Monoamine oxidase is an enzyme system responsible for breaking down purines.
3. _______ The antianxiety drug diazepam (Valium) is also used as an anticonvulsant.
4. _______ Antidepressant drugs may be used in the treatment of depression accompanied by anxiety.
5. _______ Antianxiety drugs must never be abruptly discontinued.
6. _______ There are no drugs available to relieve the symptoms of tardive dyskinesia.
7. _______ The blood pressure need not be taken during a physical assessment prior to starting therapy with a psychotherapeutic drug.
8. _______ The deltoid muscle is recommended for IM administration of a psychotherapeutic drug.
9. _______ The sedated patient should be assisted with ambulatory activities.
10. _______ Adverse reactions that may be seen with the administration of psychotherapeutic drugs are never serious.
11. _______ Behavioral records help the physician plan therapy for the patient taking a psychotherapeutic drug.

II. MULTIPLE CHOICE QUESTIONS

Circle the letter of the most appropriate answer.

1. Monoamine oxidase inhibitors are used for the treatment of _______.
   a. depression
   b. anxiety
   c. the manic phase of manic-depression
   d. nausea and vomiting associated with anxiety
2. While taking a monoamine oxidase inhibitor, the patient must not eat foods containing _______.
   a. purines b. carbohydrates c. tyramine d. fats
3. Fluoxetine (Prozac) is used in the management of _______.
   a. anxiety b. depression c. nervousness

4. When higher doses of some of the antipsychotic drugs are administered, the physician may prescribe _______ to reduce the possibility of the occurrence of parkinsonlike symptoms.
   a. cortisone
   b. a nonsteroidal anti-inflammatory drug
   c. epinephrine
   d. an antiparkinsonism drug
5. Tardive dyskinesia may occur with the use of some antipsychotic agents and is characterized by _______.
   a. a dramatic increase in urinary output
   b. rhythmic involuntary movements of the face, tongue, mouth, or jaw
   c. an inability to walk
   d. dizziness, vertigo, ataxia

Clinical Situation I

Mr. Ames is receiving chlordiazepoxide (Librium), which is an antianxiety drug.

6. Antianxiety drugs are also called _______.
   a. tranquilizers
   b. mood elevators
   c. sedatives
7. Antianxiety drugs are believed to act on subcortical areas such as the _______.
   a. thalamus and hippocampus
   b. limbic system and reticular formation
   c. medulla and spinal ganglia
   d. hypothalamus and thalamus
8. The most common adverse reactions Mr. Ames may experience with his drug are _______.
   a. nausea and vomiting
   b. diarrhea and abdominal cramping
   c. ataxia and dysuria
   d. drowsiness and sedation
9. Long-term use of this drug may result in _______.
   a. drug intolerance
   b. physical drug dependence
   c. an increasing degree of sedation
   d. anxiety

Clinical Situation II

Mrs. Lyons has had varying degrees of depression for the past 7 years. She has recently been admitted to the psychiatric unit for re-evaluation of her depression and therapy.

10. Mrs. Lyons is seen by a psychiatrist and prescribed amitriptyline (Elavil), a tricyclic antidepressant. This group of drugs _______.
    a. enhances the activity of epinephrine
    b. depletes dopamine stores in the basal ganglia
    c. blocks the reuptake of endogenous norepinephrine
11. The most common adverse reactions Mrs. Lyons may experience are _______.
    a. constipation and abdominal cramps
    b. bradycardia and double vision
    c. sedation and dry mouth
12. Observation of Mrs. Lyons' behavior will be necessary since _______.
    a. an adjustment in drug dosage may be required
    b. these drugs are rarely effective
13. Predischarge teaching of Mrs. Lyons should include which one of the following facts? _______
    a. These drugs are physically addicting; do not take longer than 8 weeks.
    b. Decrease the dose if drowsiness is severe.
    c. Increase the dose by 1 tablet if severe depression occurs.
    d. Do not drink alcoholic beverages unless use is approved by the physician.

Clinical Situation III

Mr. Howard is manic-depressive and is being given lithium.

14. Adverse reactions to lithium are toxic drug effects related to the dosage of the drug. During therapy Mr. Howard will have _______.
    a. frequent episodes of lithium toxicity
    b. periodic serum lithium levels
    c. renal function studies to determine the effects of lithium on the kidney
15. Which of the following may indicate early lithium toxicity? _______
    a. constipation, abdominal cramps, rash
    b. stupor, oliguria, hypertension
    c. nausea, vomiting, diarrhea
    d. dry mouth, blurred vision, difficulty swallowing

16. Patients receiving lithium must be _______.
   a. encouraged to drink at least 3000 mL of fluid a day
   b. given a diet low in foods containing tyramine
   c. warned not to use excess salt in their diet
   d. told to limit their fluid intake

III. FILL-IN AND ESSAY QUESTIONS

Read each of the following questions carefully and place your answer in the space provided.

1. Briefly explain why the nurse plays an important role in the administration of psychotherapeutic drugs to the hospitalized patient.

____

____

____

____

____

____

2. Why must care be exercised in giving an oral psychotherapeutic drug to a patient?

____

____

____

____

35

Drugs Used for Allergic and Respiratory Disorders

The following questions are concerned with the contents of Chapter 35, **Drugs Used for Allergic and Respiratory Disorders**.

I. TRUE OR FALSE

Read each statement carefully and place your answer in the space provided.

1. _____ Histamine is a substance manufactured by the spleen.
2. _____ Histamine is produced in response to injury.
3. _____ Some antihistamines have an antiemetic effect.
4. _____ Antihistamines are used in the treatment of allergies and therefore an allergy to these drugs does not occur.
5. _____ The use of alcohol is avoided when taking an antihistamine.
6. _____ Some bronchodilators are administered by means of an aerosol inhalator.
7. _____ Antitussives are only used when the cough produces sputum.
8. _____ An antitussive may be one of the ingredients in a nonprescription cough preparation.
9. _____ Expectorants increase the production of respiratory secretions.
10. _____ The patient's lungs are auscultated immediately before as well as after administration of a mucolytic.

II. MULTIPLE CHOICE QUESTIONS

Circle the letter of the most appropriate answer.

1. Antihistamines _____.
   a. block the action of histamine in mast cells
   b. decrease the amount of histamine produced by mast cells
   c. inactivate histamine in the liver
   d. compete for histamine at histamine receptor sites
2. The most common adverse reactions seen with administration of some of the antihistamines are _____.
   a. nausea and vomiting
   b. drowsiness and sedation
   c. abdominal cramps and constipation
   d. nasal congestion and headache

3. A bronchodilator is used to __a__.
   a. relieve bronchospasm
   b. reduce respiratory secretions
   c. increase the respiratory rate
   d. decrease the amount of air entering the lungs
4. A decongestant may be used to __c__.
   a. relieve congestion in the lungs
   b. reduce the viscosity of respiratory secretions
   c. enhance drainage of the sinuses
   d. encourage nasal secretions
5. Decongestants produce localized __b__.
   a. vasodilatation b. vasoconstriction
6. Adverse reactions seen with the administration of a sympathomimetic bronchodilator include __d__.
   a. hypotension, nausea, lightheadedness
   b. bradycardia, headache, sedation
   c. drowsiness, hypoglycemia, decreased respiratory rate
   d. rise in blood pressure, anxiety, cardiac dysrhythmias
7. When bronchospasm occurs there is a(n) __b__.
   a. increase in the amount of air reaching the lungs
   b. decrease in the lumen of the bronchi
   c. increase in the lumen of the bronchi
   d. decrease in positive pressure in the thorax
8. Which of the following show that the administration of a bronchodilator has been effective? __d__
   a. secretions are increased
   b. sputum is less viscous
   c. the patient appears sedated
   d. breathing has improved
9. If GI upset occur, the bronchodilators may be __a__.
   a. taken with food
   b. given between meals
   c. given on an empty stomach
10. Overuse of a topical decongestant may __c__.
    a. result in hypotensive episodes
    b. decrease sinus drainage
    c. cause rebound nasal congestion
    d. dilate capillaries in the nasal mucosa
11. A centrally acting antitussive __d__.
    a. anesthetizes stretch receptors in the lungs
    b. depresses the cough center in the bronchi
    c. is a narcotic that acts on the higher centers of the brain
    d. depresses the cough center in the medulla
12. Depression of the cough reflex can result in a(n) __c__.
    a. increase in the respiratory rate
    b. decrease in the viscosity of the sputum
    c. pooling of secretions in the lungs
13. A mucolytic is a drug that __d__ x b
    a. decreases respiratory secretions
    b. reduces the viscosity of respiratory secretions
    c. increases the respiratory rate
    d. aids in the production of mucus
14. An expectorant aids in __b__.
    a. decreasing the amount of secretions in the respiratory passages
    b. raising thick, tenacious secretions from the respiratory passages

III. FILL-IN AND ESSAY QUESTIONS

Read each of the following questions carefully and place your answer in the space provided.

1. Name any five uses of the antihistamines.
   1. Relief cough & cold due to allergy
   2. Treatment for Parkinson
   3. Sedation
   4. allergi conjuctive
   5. allergi rhinitis

2. Describe or list any five points that could be included in a teaching plan for the patient prescribed a bronchodilator.

1. ______________________________

____

2. ______________________________

____

3. ______________________________

____

4. ______________________________

____

5. ______________________________

____

36

Drugs Used in the Management of Gastrointestinal Disorders

The following questions are concerned with the contents of Chapter 36, **Drugs Used in the Management of Gastrointestinal Disorders**.

I. TRUE OR FALSE

Read each statement carefully and place your answer in the space provided.

1. _______ Antacids neutralize or reduce the acidity of gastric contents.
2. _______ Bulk-forming laxatives are digestible.
3. _______ Emollient laxatives soften the stool.
4. _______ Emetics are used in some cases of poison ingestion.
5. _______ Antacids impair the absorption of some drugs.
6. _______ Antidiarrheal drugs may cause drowsiness.
7. _______ Irritant or stimulant laxatives increase peristalsis by direct action on the intestine.
8. _______ Gallstone-solubilizing agents are effective for all types of gallstones.
9. _______ When ipecac is administered for poison ingestion, vomiting may be expected to occur in 2 to 3 hours.
10. _______ The long-term use of laxatives is safe and rarely causes problems.

II. MULTIPLE CHOICE QUESTIONS

Circle the letter of the most appropriate answer.

1. Anticholinergics _______.
   a. reduce gastric acidity and increase gastric motility
   b. hasten emptying of the stomach
   c. inactivate acid-secreting cells of the stomach
   d. reduce gastric motility and decrease the amount of acid secreted by the stomach
2. Pancreatic enzymes are responsible for the _______.
   a. change of starches to fats and proteins
   b. emulsification of fats and starches
   c. changing of complex sugars to glucose
   d. breakdown of fats, starches, and proteins
3. Ipecac causes vomiting because it _______.
   a. depresses the vomiting center of the medulla
   b. decreases gastric motility
   c. is irritating to the stomach
   d. increases intestinal peristalsis

4. Histamine H_2 antagonists inhibit the action of histamine _______.
   a. in the mast cells of the capillaries
   b. at histamine H_2 receptor cells in the stomach
   c. in the small intestine
   d. at histamine H_2 receptor cells in the jejunum
5. Fecal softener laxatives _______.
   a. promote water retention in the fecal mass
   b. break up the fecal mass
   c. increase intestinal peristalsis
   d. decrease intestinal peristalsis
6. Digestive enzymes may be prescribed for _______.
   a. indigestion
   b. replacement therapy in those with a peptic ulcer
   c. those with fat intolerance
   d. replacement therapy in those with pancreatic enzyme insufficiency
7. An emetic must not be given if the individual has swallowed _______.
   a. an overdose of barbiturates within the past 5 minutes
   b. paint thinner
   c. an overdose of a tranquilizer within the past 10 minutes
   d. copious amounts of a salt solution
8. A laxative may be ordered for which of the following reasons? _______
   1. to prevent straining at stool when this is contraindicated
   2. as preparation for abdominal surgery
   3. as preparation for gastroscopy
   4. as preparation for barium studies of the large intestine
   5. as preparation for an EEG

   a. 1, 2, 3 b. 1, 2, 4 c. 2, 3, 4 d. 2, 4, 5
9. Antacids containing magnesium may have a _______.
   a. constipating effect b. laxative effect
10. The antidiarrheal drug diphenoxylate (Lomotil) has drug-dependence potential; therefore _______ has been added to discourage abuse.
    a. atropine
    b. epinephrine
    c. magnesium silicate
    d. triethylene chloride
11. Laxative use may result in _______.
    a. dehydration, sodium retention
    b. potassium loss, sodium retention
    c. electrolyte imbalances, water loss
    d. fluid overload, hyperkalemia
12. Antacid tablets are _______.
    a. swallowed whole
    b. chewed before they are swallowed
13. Dry mouth, blurred vision, and urinary retention may occur with the use of _______.
    a. laxatives
    b. antacids
    c. histamine H_2 antagonists
    d. anticholinergics
14. Antidiarrheal drugs are usually given _______.
    a. twice a day, in the morning and evening
    b. hourly until diarrhea ceases
    c. after each loose bowel movement
15. Cimetidine (Tagamet) is given _______.
    a. immediately before or with meals
    b. between meals
16. Administration of a bulk-producing laxative _______.
    a. requires the patient to eat a soft diet for an optimum laxative effect
    b. is followed by enemas until clear
    c. requires the limiting of fluids until a stool is passed
    d. is followed by a full glass of water

III. FILL-IN AND ESSAY QUESTIONS

Read each of the following questions carefully and place your answer in the space provided.

1. What materials and/or equipment is made readily available when an emetic is given?

   ____

   ____

2. Briefly explain what a "laxative habit" is and why this problem occurs.

   ____

   ____

   ____

37

Antiemetic and Antivertigo Drugs

The following questions are concerned with the contents of Chapter 37, **Antiemetic and Antivertigo Drugs**.

I. TRUE OR FALSE

Read each statement carefully and place your answer in the space provided.

1. _______ An antiemetic drug is used to treat or prevent nausea or vomiting.
2. _______ Exposure to radiation may cause nausea and vomiting.
3. _______ Antiemetic drugs acting on the CTZ (chemoreceptor trigger zone) are more effective for motion sickness than those acting on the vestibular apparatus.
4. _______ Antiemetic drugs may be given prior to the administration of an antineoplastic drug.
5. _______ When used for nausea accompanying motion sickness, an antiemetic is taken approximately 2 hours after travel has started.

II. MULTIPLE CHOICE QUESTIONS

Circle the letter of the most appropriate answer.

1. Vomiting often occurs because of stimulation of the _______.
   a. stomach and its nerve supply
   b. cortex of the brain
   c. chemoreceptor trigger zone
2. Which of the following are actions of the antiemetics? _______
   1. depression of the sensitivity of the vestibular apparatus
   2. inhibition of the CTZ
   3. stimulation of the CTZ
   4. stimulation of the vestibular apparatus

   a. 1, 2　　b. 1, 3　　c. 1, 3　　d. 2, 4
3. An antiemetic may be given immediately prior to surgery to prevent _______.
   a. vomiting immediately before the anesthetic is given
   b. vertigo that occurs with the administration of a narcotic
   c. respiratory depression due to administration of a narcotic
   d. vomiting during the immediate postoperative period
4. Antivertigo drugs are _______.
   a. used for disturbances and diseases of the inner ear which cause vertigo
   b. of no value in treating nausea and vomiting

5. Stimulation of the vestibular apparatus results in _______.
   a. vertigo
   b. decreased stimulation of the CTZ
   c. decreased stimulation of higher brain centers
6. A common adverse reaction associated with the antiemetics is _______.
   a. nausea
   b. constipation
   c. vertigo
   d. varying degrees of drowsiness
7. If vomiting is severe, the blood pressure, pulse, and respiratory rate should be monitored _______.
   a. every 2 to 4 hours
   b. every 8 hours
   c. daily
8. Dehydration may occur with severe vomiting. Signs of dehydration include _______.
   1. edema
   2. poor skin turgor
   3. dry mucous membranes
   4. confusion
   5. increased urinary output

   a. 1, 2, 4 b. 1, 4, 5 c. 2, 3, 4 d. 2, 3, 5

III. FILL-IN AND ESSAY QUESTIONS

Read each of the following questions carefully and place your answer in the space provided.

1. List or describe any two points or areas that would be included in a teaching plan for the patient who has been prescribed an antiemetic.

   1. ____

   ____

   2. ____

   ____

38

Heavy Metal Compounds and Heavy Metal Antagonists

The following questions are concerned with the contents of Chapter 38, **Heavy Metal Compounds and Heavy Metal Antagonists**.

I. TRUE OR FALSE

Read each statement carefully and place your answer in the space provided.

1. _______ Silver compounds have a bactericidal effect.
2. _______ Adverse reactions to gold compounds are rarely serious.
3. _______ Stains on the skin due to the application of silver nitrate can be removed easily with soap and water.
4. _______ Improvement is almost always rapid when gold compounds are used in the treatment of rheumatoid arthritis.
5. _______ Silver sulfadiazine (Silvadene) is applied with a sterile gloved hand.
6. _______ Pain in the joints may occur for a few days following the injection of a gold compound.

II. MULTIPLE CHOICE QUESTIONS

Circle the letter of the most appropriate answer.

1. Gold compounds _______.
   a. suppress or prevent the inflammatory reactions of rheumatoid arthritis
   b. relieve the pain of osteoarthritis
   c. reverse the deformities seen with arthritis
2. The greatest benefits of the gold compounds are seen when they are _______.
   a. given for 3 consecutive weeks
   b. given twice daily for 7 days
   c. used when the disease is in remission
   d. used in the early active stages of the disease
3. Silver compounds are used as _______.
   a. systemic antibacterial agents
   b. topical antiseptics

4. Silver nitrate may be instilled into the eyes of the newborn for _______.
   a. treatment of postnatal staphylococcus eye infections
   b. prevention and treatment of gonorrheal eye infection
   c. removal of mucus
   d. treatment of syphilis
5. Silver sulfadiazine is used in the _______.
   a. eyes of the newborn to prevent staphylococcus infections
   b. prevention and treatment of infection in second- and third-degree burns
   c. treatment of eye infections resistant to other drugs
6. When using silver nitrate it must be remembered that this drug _______.
   a. has many toxic effects
   b. can only be applied twice a day
   c. will permanently stain inanimate objects
   d. cannot be applied to infected areas
7. A chelating agent is one that _______.
   a. chemically bonds metal ions, thus aiding in their elimination from the body
   b. oxidizes metals to harmless substances
   c. interferes with the absorption of heavy metals in the intestine
8. Which of the following patients may have heavy metal poisoning? The child or adult who _______.
   1. received multiple blood transfusions
   2. was exposed to large amounts of various insecticides
   3. was found eating paint chips
   4. is diagnosed as having Wilson's disease
   5. eats fish caught in water contaminated with industrial wastes

   a. 1, 2, 5, b. 2, 3, 4 c. 3, 4, 5 d. all of these
9. Penicillamine _______.
   a. has few adverse reactions when taken as directed
   b. is taken on an empty stomach
   c. is used for the treatment of lead poisoning
   d. must be taken with food

Clinical Situation

Miss Wagner, age 34, has rheumatoid arthritis.

10. Miss Wagner is given a gold compound. Adverse reactions to the gold compounds _______.
    a. usually occur after the first or second injection
    b. may occur many months after therapy is discontinued
11. Adverse reactions to the gold compounds include dermatitis, a skin reaction that is often preceded by _______.
    a. nausea
    b. diarrhea
    c. epigastric burning
    d. pruritus
12. Another adverse reaction to the gold compounds is stomatitis, which may be preceded by _______.
    a. a metallic taste
    b. a skin rash
    c. diarrhea
    d. nausea
13. Initial assessments of Miss Wagner would include _______.
    1. questioning Miss Wagner to find the cause of her arthritis
    2. examination of the areas affected by rheumatoid arthritis
    3. asking which foods make her pain worse
    4. an evaluation of her ability to carry out ADL

    a. 1, 4 b. 1, 3 c. 2, 4 d. 3, 4
14. Miss Wagner will be receiving aurothioglucose (Solganal), which is given IM. When preparing this drug for injection, it should _______.
    a. be warmed to body temperature to make it easier to withdraw the drug from the ampule
    b. be refrigerated until ready for administration
    c. not be shaken or disturbed before withdrawing the drug from the ampule

III. FILL-IN AND ESSAY QUESTIONS

Read each of the following questions carefully and place your answer in the space provided.

1. List at least three points or areas that would be included in a teaching plan for the patient receiving gold therapy as an outpatient.

   1. ______________________________

   2. ______________________________

   3. ______________________________

2. Name any four heavy metals that can be treated with a heavy metal antagonist when present in the body in excess levels.

   1. ______________________________
   2. ______________________________
   3. ______________________________
   4. ______________________________

3. List or describe any four nursing tasks or observations that should be performed when a hospitalized patient is receiving a heavy metal antagonist.

   1. ______________________________

   2. ______________________________

   3. ______________________________

   4. ______________________________

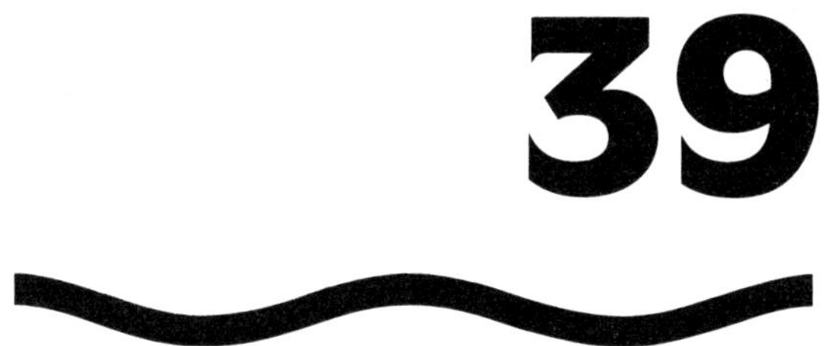

Vitamins; Drugs Used in the Treatment of Anemias

The following questions are concerned with the contents of Chapter 39, **Vitamins; Drugs Used in the Treatment of Anemias**.

I. TRUE OR FALSE

Read each statement carefully and place your answer in the space provided.

1. _______ A vitamin is a substance needed for normal growth and nutrition.
2. _______ A deficiency of vitamin C results in beriberi.
3. _______ Vitamin A is stored in the cells lining the intestines.
4. _______ The absorption of vitamin A requires the presence of bile salts.
5. _______ A deficiency of vitamin D results in rickets.
6. _______ A deficiency of vitamin E is common in young children.
7. _______ When a vitamin deficiency exists, the patient's food intake should be monitored.
8. _______ Iron is a component of hemoglobin.
9. _______ Iron cannot be stored in the body.
10. _______ Oral iron salts tend to darken the color of the stool.
11. _______ Iron dextran is only given by the parenteral route.
12. _______ Fatal anaphylactic reactions have occurred with the use of iron dextran.
13. _______ Folic acid is required for the manufacture of platelets and white blood cells.

II. MULTIPLE CHOICE QUESTIONS

Circle the letter of the most appropriate answer.

1. The vitamins manufactured by the body are vitamins _______.
   a. A and D b. B and C c. D and K d. E and K
2. Vitamin C is necessary for the _______.
   a. development of teeth, bones, blood vessels
   b. manufacture of platelets, blood clotting factors
   c. metabolism of proteins, carbohydrates, and fats

3. Situations that may require additional vitamin C are _______.
   1. diseases affecting the blood clotting mechanism
   2. pregnancy
   3. mental illnesses
   4. major surgery

   a. 1, 2 b. 1, 3 c. 2, 3 d. 2, 4
4. Vitamin B_1 plays an important role in _______.
   a. tissue respiration
   b. carbohydrate metabolism
   c. metabolism of calcium
   d. fat metabolism
5. Which of the following may have a vitamin B_1 deficiency? The _______.
   1. elderly patient
   2. chronic alcoholic
   3. postoperative patient
   4. chronically ill patient

   a. 1, 2 b. 1, 4 c. 2, 3 d. all of these
6. Which of the following may indicate a deficiency of vitamin B_2? _______
   1. bleeding tendencies
   2. changes in the cornea of the eye
   3. hair loss
   4. cheilosis
   5. glossitis

   a. 1, 2, 3 b. 1, 4, 5 c. 2, 4, 5 d. 3, 4, 5
7. Deficiencies of the vitamins B_5 and B_6 are _______.
   a. rare
   b. commonly seen in young children
   c. more likely to occur in those with a vitamin B_{12} deficiency
8. Niacin is converted by the body to _______.
   a. ascorbic acid
   b. vitamin B_3
   c. nicotinamide
9. Administration of niacin may result in _______.
   a. constipation
   b. bleeding tendencies
   c. severe generalized flushing and itching of the skin
   d. generalized edema
10. Niacin may be used to _______.
    a. increase the amount of vitamin K manufactured by the body
    b. lower blood cholesterol
    c. raise triglyceride levels
    d. counteract the effects of the water-soluble vitamins
11. Taking excessive doses of one or more water-soluble vitamins is of no value because these vitamins _______.
    a. are found in all foods
    b. are not stored in the body
    c. are extremely toxic
    d. can only be of value if the patient is chronically ill
12. Vitamin A is necessary for the _______.
    a. eye to adapt to night vision
    b. clotting of blood
    c. building of bones and teeth
    d. metabolism of calcium and magnesium
13. Vitamin D _______.
    a. regulates tissue respiration
    b. regulates protein, fat, and carbohydrate metabolism
    c. promotes intestinal absorption of calcium and phosphorus
14. Vitamin K is _______.
    a. used by the intestines to enhance calcium absorption
    b. required for the manufacture of red blood cells
    c. a catalyst in phosphorus metabolism
    d. needed by the liver to manufacture prothrombin
15. If a patient is receiving anticoagulant therapy and has an elevated prothrombin time and evidence of bleeding, the physician may prescribe _______.
    a. vitamin D
    b. vitamin A
    c. phytonadione (Mephyton)
    d. folic acid
16. Vitamin A deficiency may be seen in those with _______.
    1. colitis
    2. thrombocytopenia
    3. hepatic cirrhosis
    4. vitamin C deficiency
    5. pancreatic disease

    a. 1, 2, 4 b. 1, 3, 5 c. 2, 3, 4 d. 2, 5

17. Which one of the following may have a vitamin D deficiency? The individual _______.
   a. on renal dialysis
   b. with a potassium deficiency
   c. getting too much sunlight
   d. with hypercalcemia
18. The use of mineral oil is avoided when fat-soluble vitamins are used, because this drug may _______.
   a. break down these vitamins into useless substances
   b. prevent the absorption of these vitamins
   c. increase the absorption rate of these vitamins
19. Iron-deficiency anemia occurs when there is a _______.
   a. loss of iron from red blood cells but iron stores remain adequate
   b. loss of iron that is greater than the available iron stored in the body
20. Folic acid is required for the _______.
   a. storage of iron in the liver
   b. manufacture of platelets
   c. manufacture of red blood cells in the bone marrow
   d. storage of iron in hemoglobin
21. Which one of the following is necessary for the absorption of vitamin B_{12}? _______
   a. the extrinsic factor
   b. calcium
   c. vitamin D
   d. the intrinsic factor
22. A deficiency of vitamin B_{12} results in _______.
   a. iron-deficiency anemia
   b. microblastic anemia
   c. pernicious anemia
   d. thrombocytopenia
23. When leucovorin is given following the administration of methotrexate, it is absolutely essential that the leucovorin be given at the exact prescribed time to _______.
   a. allow a high dose of methotrexate to remain in the body for only a short time
   b. bind to the methotrexate and delay its excretion

III. FILL-IN AND ESSAY QUESTIONS

Read each of the following questions carefully and place your answer in the space provided.

1. The water-soluble vitamins are vitamins __B__ and __C__.
2. The fat-soluble vitamins are vitamins __A__, __D__, __E__, and __K__.
3. List any three points of information that may be included in a teaching plan for the patient taking iron salts for anemia.
   1. Take this drug on an empty stomach c̄ water
   2. Do not take other drugs (prescription or nonprescription) at the same time or 2 hours before or after taking iron without
   3. this drug may cause darken of the stools, constipation or diarrhea.
4. Isotretinoin (Accutane) may be prescribed for the treatment of acne. Briefly explain the danger associated with the use of isotretinoin by women.

The high risk of fetal deformities of woman that are pregnant or may become pregnant

40

Immunologic Agents

The following questions are concerned with the contents of Chapter 40, **Immunologic Agents**.

I. TRUE OR FALSE

Read each statement carefully and place your answer in the space provided.

1. _______ An antigen is formed when an antibody enters the body.
2. _______ Specific antibodies are formed for specific antigens.
3. _______ The life span of an antibody varies.
4. _______ Toxins cannot be attenuated (weakened).
5. _______ Vaccines are only given to infants.

II. MULTIPLE CHOICE QUESTIONS

Circle the letter of the most appropriate answer.

1. Antibody-producing tissues _______ distinguish between live and attenuated antigens.
   a. can
   b. cannot
2. Vaccines contain _______.
   a. only live antigens
   b. attenuated or killed antigens
   c. only killed antigens
3. Immune globulins _______.
   a. act like antibodies and antitoxins
   b. are required for the manufacture of antibodies
   c. are found in the bone marrow
   d. contain antibodies
4. Naturally acquired active immunity is attained when the individual _______.
   a. receives a vaccine containing attenuated antibodies
   b. receives a vaccine containing killed antigens
   c. develops the disease and forms antibodies against the disease
   d. forms antibodies after receiving live antigens
5. Artifically acquired active immunity is attained when the individual _______.
   a. is given a vaccine containing a killed or attenuated antigen which stimulates the formation of antibodies
   b. develops the disease and forms antibodies against the disease
   c. is given an antitoxin
6. Passive immunity is attained when the individual is given a(n) _______.
   a. toxin
   b. antigen
   c. combination of antigens and antibodies
   d. antitoxin

7. The administration of hepatitis B immune globulin is an example of ______ immunity.
   a. active
   b. naturally acquired
   c. passive
   d. artificially acquired

III. FILL-IN AND ESSAY QUESTIONS

Read each of the following questions carefully and place your answer in the space provided.

1. Define the following terms.

   Antigen. ____

   ____

   Antibody. ____

   ____

   Toxin. ____

   ____

   Antitoxin. ____

   ____

   Toxoid. ____

   ____

IV. DISCUSSION

1. Discuss the advantages and disadvantages of an immunization program for children as well as adults.* Suggestions for areas or topics that may be discussed include:
   - Is an immunization program really essential? If so, why?
   - Should some vaccines not be given, and if so which ones?
   - Should individuals who develop serious and permanent injury following administration of a vaccine be compensated?
   - Should any limit be placed on monetary compensation for the victim or her or his family?
   - What might be the consequences of holding the manufacturers of vaccines accountable for injury due to the use of a vaccine (e.g., cost, discontinuation of the vaccine)?

*Additional reading may be necessary to discuss this issue.

41

Anesthetic Agents

The following questions are concerned with the contents of Chapter 41, **Anesthetic Agents**.

I. TRUE OR FALSE

Read each statement carefully and place your answer in the space provided.

1. _______ When a general anesthetic is given, the patient loses consciousness.
2. _______ A sedative may be given with a local anesthetic.
3. _______ Prior to general anesthesia, one or more drugs may be given as part of the preanesthetic medication.
4. _______ A topical anesthetic agent must never be applied when a local anesthetic agent is to be injected.
5. _______ The general physical condition of the patient may determine the choice of general anesthetic agents.

II. MULTIPLE CHOICE QUESTIONS

Circle the letter of the most appropriate answer.

1. The rationale for use of a preanesthetic agent to dry secretions of the upper respiratory tract is _______.
   a. some gas anesthetics are irritating to the respiratory tract
   b. these drugs lessen nausea during and after surgery
   c. intravenous anesthetics increase respiratory secretions
2. The type of drug usually used to dry secretions of the upper respiratory tract is a _______ drug.
   a. cholinergic
   b. cholinergic blocking
   c. adrenergic
   d. adrenergic blocking
3. A tranquilizer with antiemetic properties may also be used as one of the preanesthetic agents. This type of drug, when given with a narcotic, usually requires _______.
   a. an increase in the dose of narcotic
   b. a decrease in the dose of the narcotic
   c. giving the tranquilizer 20 minutes before the narcotic
   d. giving the tranquilizer 30 minutes after the narcotic
4. Stage ____ is the stage of surgical analgesia.
   a. I b. II c. III d. IV
5. The type of drugs usually used for the induction of anesthesia are the _______.
   a. volatile gasses
   b. tranquilizers
   c. short-acting intravenous barbiturates
6. An endotracheal tube may be inserted to _______.
   a. administer intravenous anesthetics
   b. prevent the patient from swallowing during anesthesia
   c. keep the patient's mouth open
   d. maintain an adequate airway

7. The endotracheal tube is removed _______.
   a. during deep anesthesia
   b. once the swallowing and gag reflexes return
   c. once the patient is in Stage II of anesthesia
8. Ketamine (Ketalar) is a rapid-acting general anesthetic which produces an anesthetic state characterized by _______.
   a. severe respiratory depression
   b. bradycardia
   c. profound analgesia
   d. amnesia
9. The onset of action of the skeletal muscle relaxants is _______.
   a. rapid b. slow
10. Skeletal muscle relaxants may be used during general anesthesia to _______.
    1. facilitate insertion of an endotracheal tube
    2. assist in the removal of an endotracheal tube
    3. produce skeletal muscle relaxation during certain types of surgeries
    4. improve patient breathing after surgery

    a. all of these b. 1, 3 c. 2, 3 d. 2, 4
11. Administration of Innovar, a combination of droperidol (Inapsine) and fentanyl (Sublimaze) is called _______.
    a. deep anesthesia
    b. neuroleptanalgesia
    c. light anesthesia

III. FILL-IN AND ESSAY QUESTIONS

Read each of the following questions carefully and place your answer in the space provided.

1. Give three purposes of a preanesthetic agent.
   1. ______________________________
   2. ______________________________
   3. ______________________________
2. List any two responsibilities of the nurse during the preparation of the patient for general anesthesia.
   1. ______________________________
   2. ______________________________
3. List any five responsibilities of the nurse during the immediate postanesthesia recovery period.
   1. ______________________________
   2. ______________________________
   3. ______________________________
   4. ______________________________
   5. ______________________________

42

Drugs Used in the Management of Musculoskeletal Disorders

The following questions are concerned with the contents of Chapter 42, **Drugs Used in the Management of Musculoskeletal Disorders**.

I. TRUE OR FALSE

Read each statement carefully and place your answer in the space provided.

1. ______ Aspirin has less anti-inflammatory activity than the other salicylates.
2. ______ The nonsteroidal anti-inflammatory drugs also possess analgesic and antipyretic activity.
3. ______ The corticosteroids have potent anti-inflammatory activity.
4. ______ There are few adverse reactions associated with high-dose long-term corticosteroid therapy.
5. ______ Penicillamine has few adverse reactions.

II. MULTIPLE CHOICE QUESTIONS

Circle the letter of the most appropriate answer.

1. The anti-inflammatory activity of aspirin is thought to be due to its ability to ______.
   a. affect the hypothalamus
   b. inhibit prostaglandin synthesis
   c. affect peripheral nerve fibers
   d. block sensory impulses traveling to higher centers of the brain
2. The symptoms of gout are due to ______.
   a. the deposit of urate crystals in the joints
   b. a decrease in serum uric acid levels
   c. an increase in the excretion of uric acid

3. The tranquilizer diazepam (Valium) is also used ______.
   a. in reducing inflammation in severe rheumatoid arthritis
   b. in increasing the excretion of urates in those with gout
   c. as a skeletal muscle relaxant
4. The most common adverse reactions seen with the administration of the nonsteroidal anti-inflammatory agents are related to the ______.
   a. skin and mucous membranes
   b. bone marrow
   c. GU tract
   d. GI tract
5. One potentially serious adverse reaction associated with the administration of allopurinol (Zyloprim) is ______.
   a. uremia
   b. edema which may progress to cardiac failure
   c. skin rash which may progress to serious hypersensitivity reactions
6. The most common adverse reaction seen with the use of the skeletal muscle relaxants is ______.
   a. drowsiness
   b. nausea
   c. diarrhea
   d. constipation
7. Salicylates are given ______.
   a. on an empty stomach between meals
   b. with food, milk, or a full glass of water
8. The nonsteroidal anti-inflammatory drug indomethacin (Indocin) is given ______.
   a. on an empty stomach between meals
   b. with an antacid (when prescribed), food, or milk
   c. with a half glass of water
9. Allopurinol (Zyloprim), probenecid (Benemid), and sulfinpyrazone (Anturane) are used for gout and are given ______.
   a. with or immediately after meals
   b. between meals
   c. with a half glass of water
10. When colchicine is given for an acute attack of gout, it may be administered every 1 to 2 hours ______.
    a. for 72 hours
    b. until the swelling in the joint(s) is relieved
    c. for a total of 12 doses
    d. until pain is relieved or the patient develops vomiting and/or diarrhea
11. When a corticosteroid is being given for arthritis and alternate-day therapy is used, the drug must be given ______.
    a. with food or milk
    b. on an empty stomach
    c. before 9 AM
    d. at HS
12. The patient receiving an oral or parenteral gold salt must have ______.
    a. weekly physical therapy treatments
    b. his or her mouth inspected daily for signs of ulceration of the oral mucosa
    c. his or her position changed every 4 to 6 hours
    d. daily oral care including brushing of the teeth
13. When a drug is used in the treatment of gout, ______.
    a. the patient must remain on complete bed rest
    b. the patient is encouraged to limit his or her fluid intake
    c. the drug must be given early in the morning before breakfast
    d. a liberal fluid intake must be encouraged
14. When a patient is receiving phenylbutazone (Butazolidin) or oxyphenbutazone, which of the following requires withholding the next dose and contacting the physician? ______
    1. sore throat
    2. soreness of the mouth
    3. tarry stools
    4. fever
    5. unusual bleeding or bruising

    a. 1, 2, 3 b. 2, 4, 5 c. 2, 3, 4 d. all of these
15. The reason for the answer selected for question 14 is that ______.
    a. the patient has another illness that requires treatment
    b. these are signs of bone marrow depression, an adverse reaction associated with these drugs
    c. these symptoms are totally unrelated to the drug being given and therefore require investigation

III. FILL-IN AND ESSAY QUESTIONS

Read each of the following questions carefully and place your answer in the space provided.

1. List at least two areas or facts that would be included in a teaching plan for the patient prescribed a nonsteroidal anti-inflammatory drug for an arthritic disorder.

   1. Do not take it with aspirin or any OTC

   2. Note for dark Tarry stool

2. List at least four areas or facts that would be included in a teaching plan for the patient prescribed a drug for gout.

   1. __________

   2. __________

   3. __________

   4. __________

APPENDIX

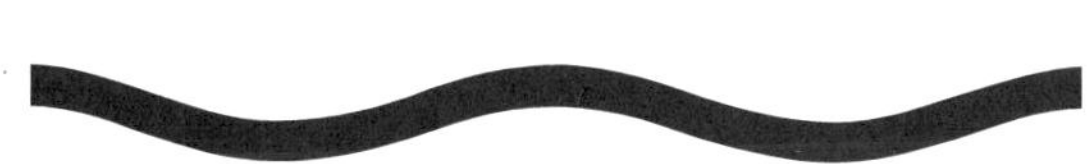

ANSWERS

CHAPTER 1

▶ ARITHMETIC REVIEW

A. FRACTIONS

1. numerator and denominator
2. a. Part of a whole; any number less than a whole.
   b. A fraction having a numerator the same as or larger than the denominator.
3. c, d, f, h, i, j
4. The numerator and denominator are not expressed in like terms

B. MIXED NUMBERS AND IMPROPER FRACTIONS

1. A whole number and a proper fraction.
2. a. 15/4 b. 5/2 c. 17/4 d. 4/3 e. 11/2 f. 17/2 g. 57/8 h. 38/3 i. 15/2 j. 23/4 k. 10/3 l. 61/3
3. a. 3 3/4 b. 5 1/4 c. 2 2/3 d. 7 1/4 e. 4 4/5 f. 11 2/3 g. 3 1/5 h. 1 1/6 i. 6 4/5 j. 5 1/3 k. 8 3/4 l. 15 1/2

C. ADDING FRACTIONS WITH LIKE DENOMINATORS

1. a. 1/2 b. 1/2 c. 1/3 d. 2/3 e. 1 f. 3/5 g. 1 h. 5/7 i. 1/2 j. 3/4 k. 1 1/3 l. 3/4 m. 11/10 or 1 1/10
2. 1/2 acre
3. a. 1 ounce b. 2/3 cup c. 1/2 cup d. 1/4 pound e. 1/16 quart f. 1/32 ounce g. 1/3 grain

D. ADDING FRACTIONS WITH UNLIKE DENOMINATORS

1. a. 11/12 b. 9/20 c. 1/2 d. 5/6 e. 7/12 f. 29/45 g. 8/15 h. 13/20 i. 1/2 j. 13/21 k. 3/64
2. 5/12 pounds

3. a. 1 1/6
   b. 1 1/2
   c. 1 2/9
   d. 1 7/15
   e. 1 11/40
   f. 1 11/21
   g. 1 9/22
   h. 1 5/8

E. ADDING MIXED NUMBERS OR FRACTIONS AND MIXED NUMBERS

1. a. 5
   b. 2 5/12
   c. 6 9/10
   d. 5 2/3
   e. 5 5/8
   f. 15 1/4
   g. 4 11/12
2. a. 15 pounds
   b. 7 1/2 pounds
   c. 4 3/4 ounces
   d. 2 1/4 pounds
   e. 3 ounces
   f. 2 1/6 ounces
   g. 1 3/4 pounds

F. COMPARISON OF FRACTIONS

1. a. 2/3
   b. 5/6
   c. 3/4
   d. 5/9
   e. 3/5
   f. 2/3
   g. 1/2
   h. 3/4
   i. 5/9
   j. 2/3
   k. 3/8
   l. 2/3
2. Mr. Burke
3. Morphine grain 1/4

G. MULTIPLYING FRACTIONS

1. a. 1/32
   b. 1/4
   c. 2/9
   d. 1/3
   e. 1/5
   f. 7/27
   g. 16/25
   h. 1/4
   i. 5/9
   j. 3/16

H. MULTIPLYING WHOLE NUMBERS AND FRACTIONS

1. a. 5/8
   b. 2 2/3
   c. 1/2
   d. 3/4
   e. 2 1/2
   f. 2 1/3
   g. 3/5
   h. 7/8
   i. 2
   j. 1
   k. 6
   l. 1
2. Mrs. Klein

I. MULTIPLYING MIXED NUMBERS

1. a. 8 1/8
   b. 12 1/4
   c. 21 25/32
   d. 8 11/14
   e. 9 9/16
   f. 11 5/32
   g. 5 1/3
   h. 8 45/48

J. MULTIPLYING A WHOLE NUMBER AND A MIXED NUMBER

1. a. 7 1/2
   b. 14
   c. 9
   d. 26 1/4
   e. 8 1/2
   f. 3 1/3
   g. 15 3/4
   h. 13 7/8
2. 20 ounces
3. 10 1/2 ounces
4. 750 milliliters
5. 10 tablets

K. DIVIDING FRACTIONS

1. a. 1/2
   b. 2/3
   c. 1 1/2
   d. 2 2/5
   e. 1/5
   f. 3/14
   g. 2
   h. 4
   i. 5 1/3
   j. 3/5
   k. 9/14
   l. 1 1/4
   m. 10
   n. 1/125
   o. 1/50
   p. 2

L. DIVIDING FRACTIONS AND MIXED NUMBERS

a. 9-1/3
b. 5
c. 2/9
d. 2-1/4
e. 4/15
f. 4-17/32
g. 16/129
h. 3/40

2. a. 7/17
   b. 5/6
   c. 11/21
   d. 2
   e. 5
   f. 2 1/16
   g. 1
   h. 7 11/15
3. a. 3
   b. 1/8
   c. 16
   d. 1/6
   e. 1/3
   f. 24
   g. 1/64
   h. 1/4
   i. 1/32
   j. 1/16
4. a. 1 1/2
   b. 1 1/3
   c. 2 2/3
   d. 5/6
   e. 1 1/4
   f. 9/10

M. RATIO

1. A way of expressing a part of a whole or the relationship of one number to another.
2. a. 1:10, 1/10
   b. 2:15, 2/15
   c. 1:5, 1/5
   d. 1:100, 1/100
   e. 1:250, 1/250
3. a. 1/1000
   b. 1/50
   c. 1/6
   d. 2/3
   e. 1/2
4. a. 1 part is to 4 parts or 1:4
   b. 1 part is to 150 parts or 1:150
   c. 1 part is to 32 parts or 1:32
   d. 1 part is to 5000 parts or 1:5000
5. 1/2 acre
6. 1/2 strength
7. weaker
8. 1/64 grain

N. PERCENT

1. parts per hundred
2. a. 32 parts per hundred
   b. 64 parts per hundred
   c. 40 parts per hundred
   d. 90 parts per hundred
   e. 20 parts per hundred
3. 84 questions were correct; 84 parts per hundred; 84/100 or 21/25
4. a. 1/4
   b. 1/2
   c. 37/100
   d. 3/4
   e. 41/100
   f. 11/50
   g. 21/25
   h. 9/10
5. a. 80%
   b. 50%
   c. 66-2/3%
   d. 62-1/2%
   e. 40%
   f. 14-2/7%
   g. 37-1/2%
   h. 25%
   i. 16-2/3%
   j. 10%
6. a. 0.2%
   b. 1%
   c. 0.1%
   d. 12-1/2%
   e. 4%
   f. 0.02%
   g. 25%
   h. 10%
   i. 0.05%
   j. 0.5%
7. a. 1:20
   b. 1:4
   c. 3:10
   d. 4:5
   e. 1:100
   f. 3:1000
   g. 2:25
   h. 3:25
8. 1:5, 1/5, 20%
9. 0.4%
10. 0.025%
11. 1:10

O. PROPORTION

1. a. 20
   b. 12
   c. 3
   d. 70
   e. 2
   f. 72
2. a. Proportion: 15 hours:1 acre::30 hours: x acres
   Solution: $x = 2$ (acres)
   b. Proportion: 15 grains:1 gram::30 grains: x grams
   Solution: $x = 2$ (grains)
   c. Proportion: 2.2 yards:1 dollar::x yards: 40 dollars
   Solution: $x = 88$ (yards)
   d. Proportion: 2.2 lbs:1 kilogram::x lbs: 40 kilograms
   Solution: $x = 88$ (pounds)
   e. Proportion: 1 share:1/60 dollar::6 shares: x dollars
   Solution: $x = 1/10$ dollar (or 10 cents)
   f. Proportion: 1 milligram:1/60 grain:: 6 milligrams:x grains
   Solution: $x = 1/10$ grain

g. Proportion: 30 milligrams:1/2 grain::90 milligrams:x grains
Solution: x = 1 1/2 grains

h. Proportion: 5 milligrams:1 kilogram:: x milligrams:64 kilograms
Solution: x = 320 milligrams

P. DECIMALS

1. A fraction in which the denominator is 10 or some power of ten.
2. a. A decimal with numbers only to the right of the decimal.
   b. A decimal with numbers to the left and right of the decimal.
3. *decimal fractions:* a. (0.01), c. (0.33), f. (0.45)
   mixed decimals: b. (1.45), d. (2.5), e. (7.5), g. (1.25)
4. a. 0.9 b. 0.04 c. 5.4 d. 0.1 e. 0.02 f. 0.001
5. a. four tenths
   b. seventy-five hundredths
   c. one and six tenths
   d. five and fifty-eight hundredths
   e. seven and seven hundred and fifty-five thousandths
6. a. 8.11 b. 4.41 c. 4 d. 24.21 e. 480.11 f. 62.327 g. 12.97 h. 68.205
7. a. 2.1 b. 53.47 c. 1.755 d. 3.875
8. a. 2.5 b. 2.5 c. 4.5 d. 21
9. a. 1.375 b. 5.28 c. 6.25 d. 7.1875 e. 18.75 f. 2.25 g. 11.8482 h. 5.25
10. a. 2.166 b. 3.5 c. 2.29 d. 5.33 e. 2.72 f. 0.9 g. 1.466 h. 1.8
11. a. 1/5 b. 13/20 c. 87/100 d. 1/2 e. 17/25

▶ THE CALCULATION OF DRUG DOSAGES

A. SYSTEMS OF MEASUREMENT

1. metric system, apothecaries' system, household measurements
2. metric system
3. gram
4. liter
5. meter
6. grains, drams, ounces
7. mimim, fluid dram, fluid ounce
8. a. mg b. kg c. ng d. mcg e. L f. mL g. cm h. m i. gr j. m̸

B. CONVERSION BETWEEN SYSTEMS

1. a. 2 g b. 2 kg c. 30 kg d. gr 1/30 e. 0.5 mL f. 1 L g. 60 mL h. 0.1 g i. 1000 mL j. 0.5 mg k. 1000 mcg l. 15 mg m. 1 mL n. 1 pt o. 2 mL p. 4 g q. 1 mg
2. a. 25 kg b. 63.63 kg c. 189.2 lb d. 23.63 kg e. 70.9 kg f. 57.27 kg

C. CONVERTING WITHIN A SYSTEM

1. a. 2 L
   b. 0.06 g
   c. 1500 mg
   d. 100 mg
   e. 3 L
   f. 500 mg
   g. 0.75 g
   h. 2 mg
   i. 200 mcg
   j. 0.5 L
   k. 1.5 L
   l. 0.5 g
   m. 2500 mg
   n. 0.1 g
   o. 0.5 mg
   p. 1500 mL

D. ORAL DOSAGES OF DRUGS

1. a. 2 tablets
   b. 2 capsules
   c. 1 tablet
   d. 1 capsule
   e. 1 tablet
   f. 2 tablets
   g. 1 capsule
   h. 3 tablets
   i. 1 tablet
   j. 1/2 tablet
   k. 2 tablets
2. a. 300 mg
   b. 600 mg
   c. 50 mg
   d. 250 mg
   e. 4 tablets
3. a. 5 mL
   b. 2 mL
   c. 10 mL
   d. 7.5 mL
   e. 2.5 mL
   f. 10 mL

E. PARENTERAL DOSAGES OF DRUGS

1. a. 1.5 mL
   b. 1 mL
   c. 1 mL
   d. 1 mL
   e. 0.5 mL
   f. 1 mL
   g. 0.5 mL (or 8 minims)
   h. 2 mL
   i. 0.5 mL
   j. 2 mL
   k. 2 mL
   l. 2 mL
   m. 0.5 mL
   n. 2.5 mL
   o. 2 mL
   p. 5 mL
2. a. 7.5 mL
   b. 2.5 mL
   c. 1. 3 mL
      2. 200,000 units
      3. 8 mL
   d. 7.5 mL

F. TEMPERATURES

1. a. 37° C
   b. 37.7° C
   c. 38.3° C
   d. 38.5° C
   e. 36.1° C
2. a. 97.1° F
   b. 86° F
   c. 101.1° F
   d. 100.4° F

G. PEDIATRIC DOSAGES

1. a. 14.54 (or 14.5) kg
   b. 1454 (or 1450) mg/kg/day
   c. 6
   d. 242 mg per dose (rounded off to nearest whole number). It should be noted that the physician, when ordering the drug, may select a dosage that is easiest to withdraw from a vial containing the reconstituted drug, therefore the dosage ordered for this child may be 250 mg per dose IV
2. a. 150 mg
   b. 50 mg
   c. 8.3 mL
3. a. 32.7 (or 33) kg
   b. 490.5 to 981 mcg; 495 to 990 mcg if weight in kilograms rounded off to nearest whole number
   c. 1000 mcg
4. 23.5 mg

H. SOLUTIONS

1. a substance dissolved in a solvent
2. 400 mL, 200 mL
3. 2 tablets, 5 tablets

CHAPTER 2
THE ADMINISTRATION OF MEDICATIONS

I. FILL-IN AND ESSAY QUESTIONS

1. the right patient, the right drug, the right dose, the right route, the right time
2. in an emergency
3. when drug is taken from the storage area, immediately before removing from the container, before returning drug to the storage area
4. oral route
5. it is difficult and dangerous to swallow when lying down
6. it helps move the drug down the esophagus into the stomach
7. intravenous, intramuscular, subcutaneous, intradermal, intralesional, intra-arterial, intra-articular, intracardiac
8. a joint
9. no, yes
10. skin and muscle
11. 45, 90
12. when the drug is highly irritating to subcutaneous tissue or will permanently stain the skin
13. almost immediately
14. above
15. true
16. creams, ointments, lotions, sprays, liquids dropped in the eyes, mists, wet dressings, liquids, creams or solids inserted/instilled in body cavities. Other answers may also be correct
17. recording the drug administered, recording information concerning administration, evaluating patient response, observing for adverse reactions. Other answers may also be correct.

II. CALCULATING IV FLOW RATES

1. a. 28–29 b. 18 c. 33–34

CHAPTER 3
GENERAL PRINCIPLES OF PHARMACOLOGY

I. TRUE OR FALSE

1. true
2. false
3. true
4. true
5. false
6. true
7. true

II. MULTIPLE CHOICE

1. b
2. a
3. c
4. a
5. d
6. b
7. d
8. a
9. c
10. b
11. a
12. d
13. c
14. a

III. FILL-IN AND ESSAY QUESTIONS

1. control of the manufacture and sale of drugs, food, and cosmetics
2. manufacture, distribution, and dispensing of drugs having a potential for abuse
3. a. 136 b. 46.6 (or 47) c. 200

CHAPTER 4
THE NURSING PROCESS AND THE ADMINISTRATION OF PHARMACOLOGIC AGENTS

I. FILL-IN AND ESSAY QUESTIONS

1. assessment, nursing diagnosis, planning, implementation, evaluation
2. identifies problems, provides a data base, may influence decisions. Other answers may also be correct.
3. information obtained during physical assessment
4. information supplied by the patient
5. to identify problems that can be solved or prevented by means of independent nursing actions
6. sorting and analyzing data, development of a patient care plan, setting goals, plan steps for carrying out nursing activities
7. carrying out a plan of action
8. preparation and administration of drugs
9. the patient's response to a drug

CHAPTER 5
PATIENT AND FAMILY TEACHING

I. TRUE OR FALSE

1. true
2. false
3. true
4. false
5. false

II. MULTIPLE CHOICE

1. b
2. a
3. c
4. c
5. c
6. a

III. FILL-IN AND ESSAY QUESTIONS

1. helps determine patient's needs and ability to learn, accept, and use information
2. answers will vary

CHAPTER 6
ADRENERGIC DRUGS

I. TRUE OR FALSE

1. true
2. false
3. false
4. true
5. true
6. false
7. true
8. true
9. true
10. false

II. MULTIPLE CHOICE

1. c
2. a
3. d
4. a
5. b
6. b
7. d
8. c
9. b
10. a
11. b
12. d

III. FILL-IN AND ESSAY QUESTIONS

1. somatic nervous system, autonomic nervous system
2. sympathomimetic drugs
3. alpha, beta

4. IV (intravenous)
5. extravasation, infiltration
6. administration of the drug by the intravenous route (invasive procedure)

CHAPTER 7
ADRENERGIC BLOCKING DRUGS

I. TRUE OR FALSE

1. false
2. true
3. true
4. true
5. false

II. MULTIPLE CHOICE

1. c
2. b
3. a
4. d
5. d
6. a
7. a
8. a
9. d

III. FILL-IN AND ESSAY QUESTIONS

1. to rise slowly from a sitting or lying position
2. on both arms in the standing, sitting, and lying positions
3. prior to the administration of the antihypertensive drug, using the same arm and position for each reading
4. see **Nursing Process**—knowledge deficit

CHAPTER 8
CHOLINERGIC DRUGS

I. TRUE OR FALSE

1. true
2. true
3. false
4. true
5. true
6. false

II. MULTIPLE CHOICE

1. d
2. c
3. a
4. d
5. a
6. c
7. b
8. d
9. b
10. c
11. d
12. b
13. a
14. b
15. c

III. FILL-IN AND ESSAY QUESTIONS

1. use cotton ball or gauze soaked in saline or other cleansing solution
2. there is some impairment of vision for a short time after insertion
3. the medication may cause a reduction in visual acuity thus increasing the risk for injury

CHAPTER 9
CHOLINERGIC BLOCKING DRUGS

I. TRUE OR FALSE

1. true
2. false
3. true
4. false
5. true
6. true
7. false
8. false

II. MULTIPLE CHOICE

1. a
2. b
3. c
4. b
5. d
6. b
7. b
8. b
9. a
10. c
11. b
12. c
13. a

III. FILL-IN AND ESSAY QUESTIONS

1. dilatation of the pupils of the eye
2. inability to focus the eyes
3. vital signs, observe for adverse drug reactions, evaluate patient's symptoms/complaints. Other answers may also be correct.
4. drug must be allowed time to produce the greatest effect on oral and upper respiratory secretions
5. see **Nursing Process**—knowledge deficit

CHAPTER 10
THE NARCOTIC ANALGESICS AND THE NARCOTIC ANTAGONISTS

I. TRUE OR FALSE

1. false
2. false
3. true
4. true
5. false
6. true
7. false
8. false
9. true
10. true

II. MULTIPLE CHOICE

1. b
2. a
3. d
4. b
5. a
6. c
7. a
8. d
9. b
10. b
11. a
12. b
13. a
14. d
15. b
16. a
17. c
18. b
19. d
20. b

III. FILL-IN AND ESSAY QUESTIONS

1. 9 to 10 AM
2. it is more important to keep the patient as comfortable as possible for the time she or he has left
3. record each bowel movement; note color, appearance, and consistency of each stool
4. see **Nursing Process**—knowledge deficit
5. answers will vary but may include feelings of abandonment, despair, anger, hostility, fear, resentment

CHAPTER 11
THE NON-NARCOTIC ANALGESICS

I. TRUE OR FALSE

1. true
2. true
3. false
4. true
5. false
6. true
7. true
8. true
9. false
10. false

II. MULTIPLE CHOICE

1. d
2. b
3. a
4. b
5. c
6. c
7. c
8. d
9. a
10. b
11. d

III. FILL-IN AND ESSAY QUESTIONS

1. 45 to 60 minutes
2. examine joints/areas involved noting their appearance, any limitation of motion, and appearance of skin over the joint; evaluate ability to carry out ADL. Other answers may also be correct.
3. see **Nursing Process**—Nursing Diagnosis
4. see **Nursing Process**—knowledge deficit

CHAPTER 12
SEDATIVES AND HYPNOTICS

I. TRUE OR FALSE

1. true
2. false
3. true
4. true
5. true
6. false
7. true
8. false
9. true
10. true

II. MULTIPLE CHOICE

1. a
2. d
3. c
4. c
5. b
6. a
7. a
8. b
9. this question is not answered as the correct answer for question number 7 is *a*
10. c

III. FILL-IN AND ESSAY QUESTIONS

1. **Sedative:** a drug producing a relaxing, calming effect
   Hypnotic: a drug that induces sleep
   Soporofic: another term for a hypnotic
2. see **Nursing Process**—Assessment
3. raise the side rails; advise patient to remain in bed and call for assistance if necessary to get out of bed
4. see **Nursing Process**—knowledge deficit

CHAPTER 13
SUBSTANCE ABUSE

I. TRUE OR FALSE

1. true
2. true
3. false
4. true
5. false
6. false
7. true
8. false
9. true
10. true
11. false
12. true

II. MULTIPLE CHOICE

1. c
2. b
3. b
4. a
5. c
6. c
7. c
8. a
9. d
10. b
11. a
12. b
13. a
14. d
15. c

III. FILL-IN AND ESSAY QUESTIONS

1. **Substance abuse:** use of a drug or chemical to produce a change in mood or behavior in a way that departs from approved medical or social patterns
   Compulsive substance abuse: a need to use any drug or chemical repeatedly to produce the desired effect
   Physical dependency: a compulsive need to use any drug or chemical substance to produce the desired effect
   Psychological dependency: a compulsion to use a substance to obtain a pleasurable experience; the mind's dependence on repeated use of a drug
2. yawning; perspiration; tearing; increased nasal discharge; gooseflesh; abdominal cramps; bone, muscle pain; nausea; vomiting; diarrhea; dilatation of the pupils; increase in temperature, pulse, respirations; intense desire for the drug
3. mental impairment; high cost; weight loss; erosion of the nasal septum; loss of job, home, savings, other possessions; malnutrition; with overdose, injury to self or others. Other answers may also be correct.
4. malnutrition, physical disease, broken marriage, loss of employment, accidents resulting in injury or death. Other answers may also be correct.

IV. DISCUSSION

1. material covered depends on individual preference; answers will vary.

CHAPTER 14
THE CARDIOTONICS AND ANTIARRHYTHMIC DRUGS

I. TRUE OR FALSE

1. true
2. false
3. true
4. true
5. false
6. false
7. false
8. true
9. true
10. true

II. MULTIPLE CHOICE

1. c
2. a
3. d
4. a
5. b
6. c
7. d
8. c
9. c
10. b
11. a
12. a
13. b
14. d
15. a

III. FILL-IN AND ESSAY QUESTIONS

1. anorexia, nausea, vomiting, diarrhea, muscle weakness, headache, apathy, drowsiness, visual disturbances, mental depression, confusion, disorientation, delerium, changes in pulse rate or rhythm. See also **Adverse Reactions Associated With the Administration of the Cardiotonics**.
2. see **Nursing Process**—Assessment
3. see **Nursing Process**—knowledge deficit
4. see **Nursing Process**—Assessment

CHAPTER 15
ANTICOAGULANT AND THROMBOLYTIC DRUGS

I. TRUE OR FALSE

1. true
2. false
3. true
4. true
5. false
6. true
7. true

II. MULTIPLE CHOICE

1. b
2. d
3. a
4. b
5. b
6. b
7. d
8. c
9. c
10. a
11. a
12. d
13. b
14. d
15. c
16. b
17. c
18. a

III. FILL-IN AND ESSAY QUESTIONS

1. urinal, bedpan, catheter drainage unit, emesis basin, nasogastric suction unit, skin, mucous membranes
2. see **Nursing Process**—knowledge deficit

CHAPTER 16
ANTIANGINAL AGENTS AND PERIPHERAL VASODILATING DRUGS

I. TRUE OR FALSE

1. true
2. true
3. true
4. false
5. false
6. true
7. true

II. MULTIPLE CHOICE

1. c
2. a
3. d
4. a
5. b
6. c
7. b
8. d
9. c
10. b

III. FILL-IN AND ESSAY QUESTIONS

1. examine area(s) for general appearance: note skin temperature; note skin color; obtain peripheral pulses
2. type of pain, whether pain radiates and to where, events that appear to cause pain, events that relieve pain
3. apply at approximately same time each day, application area must be clean and thoroughly dry before applying the system, rotate application sites. Other answers may also be correct.

CHAPTER 17
THE MANAGEMENT OF BODY FLUIDS

I. TRUE OR FALSE

1. true
2. false
3. true
4. true
5. false
6. false
7. true
8. true
9. true
10. false

II. MULTIPLE CHOICE

1. d
2. c
3. b
4. a
5. c
6. a
7. a
8. d
9. b
10. c
11. c
12. a
13. b
14. c
15. b
16. c
17. a
18. b

III. FILL-IN AND ESSAY QUESTIONS

1. see **Nursing Process**—noncompliance and knowledge deficit

CHAPTER 18
DIURETICS AND ANTIHYPERTENSIVE DRUGS

I. TRUE OR FALSE

1. true
2. false
3. true
4. false
5. true
6. true
7. false
8. true
9. false
10. true

II. MULTIPLE CHOICE

1. c
2. d
3. a
4. a
5. c
6. b
7. b
8. b
9. c
10. d
11. a
12. a
13. b
14. c
15. a

III. FILL-IN AND ESSAY QUESTIONS

1. weigh daily; intake and output; vital signs q1–4h; check areas of edema to evaluate drug effectiveness; assess general appearance, skin color, mental status
2. see **Nursing Process**—noncompliance and knowledge deficit
3. to evaluate drug response; drug dosage may require adjustment; drug may need to be discontinued or another drug added to the regimen
4. rise from a sitting or lying position slowly

CHAPTER 19
CENTRAL NERVOUS SYSTEM STIMULANTS

I. TRUE OR FALSE

1. false
2. true
3. true
4. true
5. false

II. MULTIPLE CHOICE

1. b
2. a
3. c
4. d
5. b
6. a
7. b
8. c

III. FILL-IN AND ESSAY QUESTIONS

1. blood pressure; pulse; respiratory rate, depth and pattern; assessment of patient's general condition

CHAPTER 20
INSULIN AND ORAL HYPOGLYCEMIC AGENTS

I. TRUE OR FALSE

1. true
2. true
3. true
4. false
5. true
6. true
7. false
8. true
9. true
10. false

II. MULTIPLE CHOICE

1. d
2. c
3. a
4. a
5. a
6. d
7. b
8. c
9. b
10. c
11. b
12. a
13. d
14. b
15. d
16. c

III. FILL-IN AND ESSAY QUESTIONS

1. hypoglycemia, hyperglycemia
2. see Table 21-2
3. see Table 21-2
4. dilute corn syrup; orange juice with sugar; commercial glucose products; glucagon SC, IV, IM; glucose 10% or 50% IV
5. see **Nursing Process**—knowledge deficit
6. see **Nursing Process**—knowledge deficit

CHAPTER 21
THE SULFONAMIDES

I. TRUE OR FALSE

1. true
2. false
3. true
4. true
5. false

II. MULTIPLE CHOICE

1. b
2. d
3. a
4. b
5. c
6. d
7. b
8. b
9. a

III. FILL-IN AND ESSAY QUESTIONS

1. see **Nursing Process**—knowledge deficit

CHAPTER 22
THE PENICILLINS AND THE CEPHALOSPORINS

I. TRUE OR FALSE

1. false
2. true
3. false
4. true
5. true

II. MULTIPLE CHOICE

1. d
2. b
3. a
4. c
5. b
6. c
7. b
8. a
9. a
10. c
11. b

III. FILL-IN AND ESSAY QUESTIONS

1. color and type of drainage; look for signs of redness, inflammation; determine if an odor is present; question the patient about pain or discomfort at the infected site
2. see **Nursing Process**—noncompliance and knowledge deficit

CHAPTER 23
THE BROAD-SPECTRUM ANTIBIOTICS AND ANTIFUNGAL DRUGS

I. TRUE OR FALSE

1. true
2. false
3. true
4. false
5. true
6. true
7. false
8. true

II. MULTIPLE CHOICE

1. b
2. d
3. a
4. c
5. a
6. b
7. d
8. b
9. c
10. c
11. b
12. c
13. a
14. b
15. d
16. c
17. a
18. c

III. FILL-IN AND ESSAY QUESTIONS

1. see **Nursing Process**—noncompliance and knowledge deficit
2. see **Nursing Process**—noncompliance and knowledge deficit

CHAPTER 24
ANTITUBERCULAR AND LEPROSTATIC DRUGS

I. TRUE OR FALSE

1. false
2. true
3. true
4. true
5. false
6. true

II. MULTIPLE CHOICE

1. a
2. c
3. d
4. a
5. c
6. b
7. d
8. c

CHAPTER 25
DRUGS USED IN THE TREATMENT OF PARASITIC INFECTIONS

I. TRUE OR FALSE

1. true
2. true
3. true
4. true
5. false

II. MULTIPLE CHOICE

1. c
2. d
3. a
4. c
5. b
6. a
7. b
8. d
9. c
10. d
11. b
12. b
13. a

III. FILL-IN AND ESSAY QUESTIONS

1. see **Nursing Process**—noncompliance and knowledge deficit

CHAPTER 26
MISCELLANEOUS ANTI-INFECTIVE DRUGS

I. TRUE OR FALSE

1. true
2. false
3. false
4. true
5. true
6. true
7. true
8. false
9. true
10. true

II. MULTIPLE CHOICE

1. a
2. c
3. b
4. d
5. b
6. a
7. d
8. b
9. b
10. c
11. a
12. b
13. b

III. FILL-IN AND ESSAY QUESTIONS

1. see **Nursing Process**—noncompliance and knowledge deficit
2. anxiety may be related to the diagnosis and prognosis because the drug is given to those with AIDS
3. eye infections, treatment of glaucoma, preparation for eye surgery, eye pain or inflammation, ear infection, ear pain, inflammation of the external auditory canal
4. see **Nursing Process**—knowledge deficit

IV. DISCUSSION

1. topics and responses will vary

CHAPTER 27
PITUITARY AND ADRENAL CORTICAL HORMONES

I. TRUE OR FALSE

1. false
2. true
3. true
4. false
5. false
6. true
7. false
8. true
9. false
10. true
11. true

II. MULTIPLE CHOICE

1. d	6. b	11. c	16. b
2. b	7. d	12. b	17. c
3. a	8. a	13. c	18. d
4. c	9. d	14. d	19. a
5. a	10. c	15. a	20. a

III. FILL-IN AND ESSAY QUESTIONS

1. vasopressin (antidiuretic hormone, ADH) and oxytocin
2. twice the daily dose given every other day before 9 AM. Giving the drug before 9 AM does not affect the release of ACTH and minimizes certain undesirable glucocorticoid effects
3. see **Nursing Process**—noncompliance and knowledge deficit, long-term or high-dose glucocorticoid therapy, mineralocorticoid therapy

CHAPTER 28
MALE AND FEMALE HORMONES

I. TRUE OR FALSE

1. true	3. false	5. false
2. true	4. false	

II. MULTIPLE CHOICE

1. a	5. a	9. b	13. b
2. b	6. d	10. d	14. c
3. c	7. b	11. a	
4. b	8. c	12. c	

III. FILL-IN AND ESSAY QUESTIONS

1. androgens
2. estrogen, progesterone
3. facial hair, deepening of the voice, male-pattern baldness, enlargement of the clitoris, patchy hair loss, skin pigmentation, acne
4. see **Nursing Process**—noncompliance and knowledge deficit
5. see **Nursing Process**—noncompliance and knowledge deficit
6. psychologic addiction, uncontrolled rage, severe depression, suicidal tendencies, inability to concentrate, personality changes

CHAPTER 29
THYROID AND ANTITHYROID DRUGS

I. TRUE OR FALSE

1. false	3. true	5. true
2. false	4. false	

II. MULTIPLE CHOICE

1. a	5. b	9. a	13. c
2. d	6. d	10. b	14. b
3. c	7. a	11. d	
4. c	8. d	12. d	

III. FILL-IN AND ESSAY QUESTIONS

1. see Table 29-1
2. see **Nursing Process**—noncompliance and knowledge deficit

CHAPTER 30
DRUGS ACTING ON THE UTERUS

I. TRUE OR FALSE

1. true
2. false
3. true
4. false
5. true

II. MULTIPLE CHOICE

1. c
2. a
3. d
4. b
5. a
6. b
7. d
8. c
9. a
10. b
11. b
12. c
13. b

III. FILL-IN AND ESSAY QUESTIONS

1. FHR: mother's blood pressure, pulse, respiratory rate; activity of the uterus
2. onset of labor; time interval between contractions; length and intensity of each contraction; blood pressure, pulse, respiratory rate. Additional answers may also be correct.

IV. DISCUSSION

1. responses will vary.

CHAPTER 31
ANTINEOPLASTIC DRUGS

I. TRUE OR FALSE

1. true
2. false
3. true
4. true
5. false
6. true
7. true
8. true
9. true
10. false

II. MULTIPLE CHOICE

1. a
2. b
3. b
4. c
5. d
6. c
7. a
8. a
9. d
10. d
11. c
12. b

III. FILL-IN AND ESSAY QUESTIONS

1. see **Nursing Process**—Assessment
2. see **Nursing Process**—knowledge deficit

IV. DISCUSSION

1. responses will vary.

CHAPTER 32
ANTICONVULSANT DRUGS

I. TRUE OR FALSE

1. true
2. true
3. false
4. false
5. true

II. MULTIPLE CHOICE

1. c
2. a
3. d
4. c
5. a
6. b
7. a
8. c
9. d
10. b
11. a
12. d

III. FILL-IN AND ESSAY QUESTIONS

1. see **Nursing Process**—noncompliance and knowledge deficit

CHAPTER 33
ANTIPARKINSONISM DRUGS

I. TRUE OR FALSE

1. true
2. true
3. true
4. false

II. MULTIPLE CHOICE

1. a
2. c
3. a
4. b
5. d
6. b
7. d
8. b
9. a
10. a
11. b

III. FILL-IN AND ESSAY QUESTIONS

1. see **Nursing Process**—Assessment
2. remove throw rugs, install handrail next to toilet, remove obstacles that may cause falls, injury. Other answers may also be correct.

CHAPTER 34
PSYCHOTHERAPEUTIC DRUGS

I. TRUE OR FALSE

1. true
2. false
3. true
4. true
5. true
6. false
7. false
8. false
9. true
10. false
11. true

II. MULTIPLE CHOICE

1. a
2. c
3. b
4. d
5. b
6. a
7. b
8. d
9. b
10. c
11. c
12. a
13. d
14. b
15. c
16. a

III. FILL-IN AND ESSAY QUESTIONS

1. patient response to drug therapy requires around-the-clock observation of the hospital patient, as frequent dosage adjustments may be necessary. Accurate assessments for adverse drug reactions are important when the patient communicates poorly.
2. the patient may have difficulty swallowing or may be extremely withdrawn and not swallow the drug. Other answers may also be acceptable.

CHAPTER 35
DRUGS USED FOR ALLERGIC AND RESPIRATORY DISORDERS

I. TRUE OR FALSE

1. false
2. true
3. true
4. false
5. true
6. true
7. false
8. true
9. true
10. true

II. MULTIPLE CHOICE

1. d
2. b
3. a
4. c
5. b
6. d
7. b
8. d
9. a
10. c
11. d
12. c
13. b
14. b

III. FILL-IN AND ESSAY QUESTIONS

1. see **ANTIHISTAMINES**, Uses of Antihistamines
2. see **Nursing Process**—knowledge deficit

CHAPTER 36
DRUGS USED IN THE MANAGEMENT OF GASTROINTESTINAL DISORDERS

I. TRUE OR FALSE

1. true
2. false
3. true
4. true
5. true
6. true
7. true
8. false
9. false
10. false

II. MULTIPLE CHOICE

1. d
2. d
3. c
4. b
5. a
6. d
7. b
8. b
9. b
10. a
11. c
12. b
13. d
14. c
15. a
16. d

III. FILL-IN AND ESSAY QUESTIONS

1. emesis basin, towels, specimen containers, suction machine
2. dependence on a laxative to have a bowel movement, resulting from long-term laxative use

CHAPTER 37
ANTIEMETIC AND ANTIVERTIGO DRUGS

I. TRUE OR FALSE

1. true
2. true
3. false
4. true
5. false

II. MULTIPLE CHOICE

1. c
2. a
3. d
4. a
5. a
6. d
7. a
8. c

III. FILL-IN AND ESSAY QUESTIONS

1. see **Nursing Process**—knowledge deficit

CHAPTER 38
HEAVY METAL COMPOUNDS AND HEAVY METAL ANTAGONISTS

I. TRUE OR FALSE

1. true
2. false
3. false
4. false
5. true
6. true

II. MULTIPLE CHOICE

1. a
2. d
3. b
4. b
5. b
6. c
7. a
8. d
9. b
10. b
11. d
12. a
13. c
14. a

III. FILL-IN AND ESSAY QUESTIONS

1. see **Nursing Process**—noncompliance and knowledge deficit
2. lead, iron, gold, arsenic, mercury, copper
3. see **Nursing Process**—Planning and Implementation

CHAPTER 39
VITAMINS; DRUGS USED IN THE TREATMENT OF ANEMIAS

I. TRUE OR FALSE

1. true
2. false
3. false
4. true
5. true
6. false
7. true
8. true
9. false
10. true
11. true
12. true
13. false

II. MULTIPLE CHOICE

1. c
2. a
3. d
4. b
5. d
6. c
7. a
8. c
9. c
10. b
11. b
12. a
13. c
14. d
15. c
16. b
17. a
18. b
19. b
20. c
21. d
22. c
23. a

III. FILL-IN AND ESSAY QUESTIONS

1. B and C
2. A, D, E, and K
3. see **Nursing Process**—noncompliance and knowledge deficit
4. the high risk of fetal deformities in women who are pregnant or may become pregnant

CHAPTER 40
IMMUNOLOGIC AGENTS

I. TRUE OR FALSE

1. false
2. true
3. true
4. false
5. false

II. MULTIPLE CHOICE

1. b
2. b
3. d
4. c
5. a
6. d
7. c

III. FILL-IN AND ESSAY QUESTIONS

1. **Antigen:** a foreign protein substance that enters the body
   Antibody: a protein manufactured by lymphoid tissue and the reticuloendothelial system
   Toxin: A substance produced by some bacteria
   Antitoxin: a substance that acts like antibodies and is produced in response to a toxin
   Toxoid: a weakened toxin

IV. DISCUSSION

1. topics and responses will vary

CHAPTER 41
ANESTHETIC AGENTS

I. TRUE OR FALSE

1. true
2. true
3. true
4. false
5. true

II. MULTIPLE CHOICE

1. a
2. b
3. b
4. c
5. c
6. d
7. b
8. c
9. a
10. b
11. b

III. FILL-IN AND ESSAY QUESTIONS

1. to decrease anxiety and apprehension; to dry secretions of the upper respiratory tract; to lessen the incidence of nausea and vomiting in the immediate postanesthesia recovery period
2. see section: **GENERAL ANESTHESIA**
3. see **GENERAL ANESTHESIA**, Nursing Implications

CHAPTER 42
DRUGS USED IN THE MANAGEMENT OF MUSCULOSKELETAL DISORDERS

I. TRUE OR FALSE

1. false
2. true
3. true
4. false
5. false

II. MULTIPLE CHOICE

1. b
2. a
3. c
4. d
5. c
6. a
7. b
8. b
9. a
10. d
11. c
12. b
13. d
14. d
15. b

III. FILL-IN AND ESSAY QUESTIONS

1. see **Nursing Process**—noncompliance and knowledge deficit
2. see **Nursing Process**—noncompliance and knowledge deficit